Trusting Medicine

Trusting Medicine
The Moral Costs of Managed Care

Patricia Illingworth, J.D., Ph.D.

Routledge
Taylor & Francis Group

LONDON AND NEW YORK

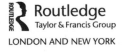

First published in 2005 by Routledge
2 Park Square, Milton Park, Abingdon. Oxfordshire OX14 4RN

Simultaneously published in the USA and Canada
By Routledge
270 Madison Avenue, New York, NY 10016, USA

Routledge is an imprint of the Taylor & Francis Group

Typeset in 10/12 Sabon by J&L Composition, Filey, North Yorkshire
Printed and bound in Great Britain by TJ International, Padstow,
Cornwall

British Library Cataloguing in Publication Data
A catalogue record for this book is available from the British Library

Library of Congress Cataloguing in Publication Data
A catalogue record has been requested

ISBN 0-415-36482-5 (hbk)
ISBN 0-415-36483-3 (pbk)

For my daughter Zoë with so much love.

Contents

Acknowledgements

This book focuses on the doctor–patient relationship and the role it plays in the health and welfare of the community. Many people have helped with this book both directly as researchers and readers and indirectly, by providing support and encouragement to me. I benefitted enormously from the comments, conversations, and suggestions of Regis de Silva, John Field, Leonard Fleck, Thomas Gutheil, Robert Hamm, Michael Hendryx, Tim Murphy, Udo Schuklenk, James Sabin, Alan Stone, Paul Ward, and Dan Wikler. I am grateful to each of them. Wendy Parmet and Margaret Somerville gave the last draft of the book a very careful reading. Their extensive comments and friendship throughout the long process of writing this book are deeply appreciated.

Much of this book was written while I was an Ethics Fellow in the Division of Medical Ethics at Harvard Medical School. I thank both Northeastern University for a much-needed sabbatical and the Division of Medical Ethics for providing me with a collegial atmosphere in which to write it. Walter Robinson ran a wonderful seminar, an intellectually rich and engaging forum, in which to think about what it is to do bioethics and to develop a research project. I am extremely grateful to him and seminar members, all of whom provided me with excellent comments on an early draft of this book. I also learned a great deal from the faculty seminar conducted by Marcia Angell and thank her for the thoughtfulness she brought to the seminar. I have also benefitted enormously from conversations with members of the Program in Psychiatry and the Law at Harvard Medical School. I thank them for always welcoming me to the program.

I have been blessed with many good friends who have supported me with their kindness, laughter, curiosity and patience throughout the process of writing this book. Although there are many friends and family members who deserve mention, I am limited to naming only a few and am particularly grateful to Claire Aldrich, Harold Burzstajn, Jillian Clare-Cohen, Nancy Dearman, Dean Gilmour, Crystal Greene, Russell, Judy and Suzanne Higley, Joan Illingworth, Martin Illingworth, Charlotte Ikels, Erika Jungblut, John Kotter, Claude Menders, Joanne Cipolla Moore, Johnathon Palmer,

Jim Peloquin, Ross Posnock, Joan Riley, Susan Schechter, Mimi Smith, Margot and Bill Usdan, and Ezra Vogel.

This book would not have been written but for the diligence of a number of outstanding research assistants who helped me locate materials, facts, and figures. Audrey Capuano, Forrester Liddle, Bronwyn Page, and most particularly Nela Suka were thoughtful, careful researchers, and always good-natured. But I owe a special debt of gratitude to Jessica Wolland who did a substantial amount of the research for this book and with whom I worked closely.

I learned a great deal from her intelligence, political commitment, and standards of excellence.

Routledge has been a very supportive press and I am grateful to Karen Bowler, Claire Gauler and Abigail Griffin for their enthusiasm, as well as their thoughtful approach to this book and Carol Ball for her excellent index.

I also wish to thank my colleagues at Northeastern University for their comments on early drafts of this material. Much appreciation goes to Michael Lipton and Stephen Nathanson, both of whom found ways to facilitate my research. I am also grateful, of course, to the many students in my bioethics classes who have discussed with me the material contained in this book. Dean Stellar has been a strong voice for interdisciplinary research at Northeastern and I thank him for that.

Finally, I'd like to thank the editors and publishers of the following articles for granting me permission to use previously published materials in this work:

Bluffing, Puffing, and Spinning in Managed-Care Organizations. *Journal of Medicine and Philosophy*, 2000; 25, No. 1: 62–76. Copyright © The Journal of Medicine and Philosophy, Inc. Reprinted by permission.

Employer Leadership in the Era of Workplace Rationing. *Cambridge Quarterly of Healthcare Ethics*, 2001; 10, No. 2: 172–183. Copyright © Cambridge Quartely Healthcare Ethics. Reprinted by permission.

Trust: The Scarcest Medical Resources. *Journal of Medicine and Philosophy*, 2002; 27, No. 1: 31–46. Copyright © The Journal of Medicine and Philosophy, Inc. Reprinted by permission.

Introduction

Most of us spend a good portion of our waking hours in the company of other people. Family, friends, neighbors, business associates, store clerks, and postal workers are among those with whom we interact on a regular basis. These relationships provide us with a number of goods and services. We purchase our groceries, turn to our neighbors for a cup of flour, interact with our children's teachers, and further our professional interests with our colleagues. However, many of these interactions also provide us with opportunities to socialize, network, and to secure much-needed human warmth and affection. Less obviously, they provide us with a social support system and a mechanism for achieving cooperative goals that are in our mutual and collective interest.

Trust is at the heart of these relationships. Without trust many people would not be willing to tend their neighbors' plants, comfort a sick relative, deliver meals on wheels to the elderly, give the benefit of the doubt to a clerk who makes a mistake, or participate in the demanding activities of the Parent Teacher Association. We are willing to undertake these activities because we trust that others will do likewise. This is called 'generalized reciprocity.' Unfortunately, social surveys reveal that Americans are less trusting today than they were in the past.

The networks of relationships and social interactions can also constitute social capital. Before proceeding, it is important to have a working definition of 'social capital.' 'Social capital' should be understood as a public good (though it is also a private good) consisting of the network of norms, activities, and values, including trust, that facilitate cooperative activity.[1] Like physical capital (books, tools, computers, etc.), and human capital (skills, knowledge, talents), social capital is productive. It can be used for the benefit of individuals, organizations, and the community. Social capital inheres in social relationships and facilitates the cooperation that is essential to make those relationships productive.[2] In this respect, social capital, and the trust that is both at its heart, and an outcome of it, is an important social resource. Social relations and social structures can be more and less conducive to the development of social capital. Parents, for example, could share their physical capital with their children, but be so preoccupied with their professional obligations that they fail to develop the social capital within the family that the child can use in other contexts.

Because relationships that are rich in trust are important for the cultivation of social capital, and the doctor–patient relationship has traditionally been rich in trust, I believe that it, as well as other healing relationships, is important for social capital. Given its importance for the cultivation of social capital, I will argue that the doctor–patient relationship deserves our protection. With the current state of our healthcare system, it should come as no surprise that the doctor–patient relationship has undergone significant changes.

Our health-care system is in distress. Costs are high; patients, providers, insurers, and employers/payers are disgruntled. Many people viewed managed care as a solution to escalating health-care costs. For a variety of reasons, however, it appears not to have fulfilled its promise over the long term to cut costs and provide increased access to high-quality health care. There has now emerged a significant backlash against managed care.[3] Many states have enacted mandates to smooth out some of the rough edges around managed care, but often, because of Employment Retirement Income Security Act (ERISA) preemption, these do not apply to the millions of people who are enrolled in self-insured employer-based plans.[4] ERISA is a federal act that applies to employee benefits, including health insurance, and has the unfortunate consequence that many state laws governing health care do not apply to ERISA health plans. Congress is entertaining the enactment of a Patients' Bill of Rights in order to remedy some of these difficulties. However, since 9/11 the nation has been largely preoccupied with security from terrorism. As we reflect on the many challenges posed by the health-care system and consider different policy responses to them, it is important that our response not be based on a narrow conception of what data and perspectives are relevant to the dialogue.

In this book, I attempt to reframe the dialogue about health care, and particularly about managed care, by looking at the consequences of managed care for the community. In the past, a good portion of the ethical analysis of managed care focused on individual patients and their right to contract with managed plans.[5] My analysis will include a discussion of this, but will also look at the doctor–patient relationship as part of the fabric of society. Although I refer most often to the 'doctor–patient relationship,' much of what I have to say applies to other providers, including nurses. Rather than restrict my discussion to the standard considerations of how health-care systems affect the individual doctor–patient relationship, I will look more deeply into the consequences of how fundamental changes in the doctor–patient relationship affect the general level of trust available to our society.

This analysis will entail making certain generalizations, for example, about the nature of the doctor–patient relationship and about patient trust. These generalizations and the studies and analysis that they are based on are limited by the fact that different populations within the United States have different experiences within the health-care system.[6] It would not be surprising to find that the differences in health care received by the poor, women, and African Americans, for example, resulted in different levels of trust as well.[7] Unfortunately, this important topic is beyond the scope of this book.

Although the considerations I take into account and the analysis I make could fruitfully be applied to a wide variety of policies and organizations, the focus of this book is on health plans that aggressively manage care. Managed medical care has rapidly come to affect a great number of people within the community. As of 2003, 95 percent of insured Americans were enrolled in some form of managed care.[8] Indeed, the magnitude of its impact on medical practice is so great that some legal scholars are now recommending changing the standard of medical care to be considered in medical malpractice.[9]

In 2001, enrollment in the most restrictive forms of managed care, health maintenance organizations (HMOs), dropped significantly for the first time since 1993, primarily in favor of more flexible kinds of managed care, such as Preferred Provider Organizations (PPOs).[10] Since then, HMO enrollment has wavered somewhat, but overall continues to decline as PPO enrollment continues to rise.[11] Although there is some evidence that this decline has stabilized, managed care continues to trouble policymakers, the media, patients, advocacy groups, politicians, and Congress.[12] Moreover, very recent surveys suggest that a managed care rebound is underway, as major health plans begin to reintroduce cost containment mechanisms once abandoned in the wake of the backlash against managed care.[13] Many criticisms have been laid against aggressively managed Medicare, some of which may be true, some exaggerations, and others may be false. However, I will focus primarily on how trust and social capital may have been affected by managed care.

Concerns have been articulated that truth telling is compromised in managed care medicine,[14] that capitation, a hallmark of managed care, adversely affects the fiduciary relationship between doctor and patient,[15] and that genuine consent to reimbursement mechanisms is implausible.[16] From the perspective of ethics and law, questions about consent are of particular interest because consent is a powerful ethical tool. Given our deference, morally, to the autonomous and self-determining actions of people, their consent to an activity, behavior, or harm to themselves, can take the moral sting out of morally problematic behavior. In medicine, this deference to individuals and their autonomy has loomed large—in part because of the cultural emphasis on autonomy, but also because medical procedures are performed on people. Consent has been needed to transform what would otherwise count as unconsented touching (assault) into consented medical procedures.[17]

A discussion about the benefits of trust from the doctor–patient relationship for the community has not been explicitly addressed by bioethics. This omission may have been fueled by the belief that many health problems are well within the control of the individuals who have them. But the quality of our social life—our interactions with each other and our community, factors often outside the control of individuals, can also influence health.[18] More recently, we have learned that the presence or absence of supportive social relations and social capital can influence health outcomes.[19] Put in the simplest terms, the quality of our social life affects our health. This will come as no surprise to many health care providers, who know very well the therapeutic power of the doctor–patient relationship.[20]

As the cost of medical care rose (through the 1980s and early 1990s), beyond what employers felt comfortable paying, health plans that manage care were more widely adopted and placed under increasing pressure by the employers/payers to lower costs.[21] Managed medical care was premised on the assumption that in order to lower costs someone other than the physician and patient would need to determine the appropriateness of care. Underlying this argument, insofar as it is a moral argument, is a justice-based concern about controlling health-care expenditures in order to make them accessible to more people. However, in order to control costs, health-care would have to be managed, and trade-offs would have to be made. Advocates of managed care appealed to a standard distributive justice argument invoking the benefits to the community (those who did not have insurance) and burdens to individuals (having their care managed). Alternatively, one could simply assert that employers/payers chose managed plans over other kinds of plans because the former promised to reduce health-care costs. Many empolyers wanted to use that money for other purposes, for example, to improve their competitive edge internationally.

Much of the dialogue about the health-care system, and specifically about managed care, has focused on costs. Yet, costs have been narrowly construed with little attention to the moral consequences of cost shifting or to externalities and the costs that do not easily translate into medical expenditure dollars. Although well intentioned, that approach can be misleading. Costs can be broader than those identified by medical expenditure calculations. For example, there can be costs to trust between doctor and patient. If we ignore these qualitatively different costs, then calculations focusing primarily on medical expenditures will not reflect the *true* costs. We will not have an accurate reflection of the costs of adopting particular reimbursement mechanisms. A more accurate picture of the costs associated with a reimbursement mechanism requires a comprehensive analysis of different kinds of costs as well as benefits.

The discussion of trust, the doctor–patient relationship, and social capital developed in this book focuses on the American health-care system. That system is unique in its whole-hearted adoption of private, market-driven health care. Yet a number of lessons can be fruitfully drawn from the analysis in this book and applied to other health-care systems. Most, if not all, of the Western industrial countries face challenges similar to those of the United States, namely, the need to control the ever-expanding health-care costs and ensure quality health care. Although the U.S. spends more on health care than any other country, it is not the only 'big spender.' In 2002, both Germany and Switzerland spent more than 10 percent of their GDP on health care.[22] Spending is also increasing in Britain where historically expenditures on health care have been held down. It has been predicted that spending on health care will reach 9.4 percent of the GDP by 2007–08, up from 6.9 percent in 1998.[23] France too has increased its spending on health care. Whether or not this spending is justified in terms of improved health outcomes, most nations are concerned about controlling escalating health-care costs and ensuring quality care.

Among the strategies countries consider using to contain spending on health care are increased competition and increased use of private insurers and providers. In Britain for example, beginning with the Griffiths Report in 1983, the National Health Service (NHS) began to explore a more business-like approach to their health-care system, with the use of internal market forces in the health-care system. In 1991, the NHS internal market reforms introduced a split between providers and purchasers.[24] More recently, the NHS introduced increased competition into the health-care system by awarding contracts for some routine operations, such as hip replacement, to foreign health-care groups. In addition, some countries already employ various kinds of managed-health strategies, whether or not these strategies are called managed-health care, and are in the process of expanding their use of these strategies. Integrated health care and managed mechanisms are used in Britain with the fundkeeper/gatekeeper system and in the Netherlands with the use of gatekeepers.[25] Government now devotes 75 percent of NHS funding to 300 local NHS Primary Care Trusts (PCTs), which function on a capitated basis.[26] Indeed, some PCTs are collaborating with U.S. managed-care plans to improve their management processes with respect to chronic diseases.[27] In Canada, capitated payment systems have begun to appear, and global caps on physician fees are present.[28] Thus, many of the strategies associated with managed care have been adopted by other developed nations, and these nations face many of the same economic challenges that may drive them to employ more aggressive versions of these strategies.

As different nations consider whether and to what extent to embrace managed health strategies, so widely adopted in the U.S., they can perhaps make a wiser choice, learning from the U.S. experience. It is vital to consider the impact of these strategies on trust between doctor and patient and, ultimately, on the welfare of the community. Of course, some nations, such as Britain and Canada, also have an historical commitment to equal access to health care that may soften some of the harsher effects of aggressively practiced managed care on trust and social capital. However, given the enormous benefits associated with social capital and the many challenges it faces in modern industrial societies, it is not clear that any nation has social capital to spare.

An overview of this book

In this book, I posit that some managed-care plans entail social costs that ought to be taken into account in a moral and policy evaluation of these plans. We have a moral duty to take into account the harm to the community from a loss of trust and social capital. My goal is not to recommend a particular reimbursement mechanism, and it is not to defend fee-for-service. Although fee-for-service and some loosely managed plans have a number of virtues with respect to facilitating trust and social capital, I also recognize that the decision about what reimbursement mechanism to implement does not hinge only on the wherewithal of the mechanism to cultivate these goods. Having said this, I shall make the case that we ought not to underestimate the importance of trust and social capital in fashioning health plans and the cost containment strategies that they adopt.

A brief 'nuts and bolts' overview of health-care spending and of some of the conceptual and ethical material used in this book is presented in Chapter 1. This provides the reader with the conceptual background against which to frame the arguments of the book. Chapter 2 looks at how some of the cost containment mechanisms used by managed care can create an environment in which the prevailing truth-telling paradigm is closer to that of corporate America than to what we have come to expect in a fiduciary context such as medicine. Not only can we expect that physicians and health plans will 'bluff, puff, and spin,' but we can also speculate that in such an environment patients may begin to manipulate information. The problem with this scenario is two-fold. First, patients put their health at risk when they deceive their physicians. Second, the conceptual apparatus that takes the moral sting out of 'bluffing, puffing, and spinning' in the organizational context, consent, does not seem to apply in the context of health-care delivery. There is good reason to believe that some of the cost containment mechanisms used by managed care will create an environment ripe for 'bluffing, puffing, and spinning.' In a medical context, practices of this kind cannot be morally justified, at least not with the same arguments used to justify them in the context of business.

In Chapter 3, I look at how 'trust' between doctor and patient fares in the context of aggressively managed medical care. The topic of trust is well traversed in health policy and bioethics, and it has resurfaced as a matter of concern as managed care has gained ground. There are a number of empirical studies showing that the trust between doctor and patient has been adversely affected by some of the cost containment mechanisms used in managed health care.[29] Although I discuss some of these studies, I also make use of a conceptual model of trust as articulated by Russell Hardin and reflected in some of the studies done by David Mechanic on medical trust. Hardin has a two-fold approach to trust. On the first, the 'encapsulated interest' account, trust is thought to follow when the person doing the trusting, the entruster, can see that it is in the interest of the trustee to be trustworthy. On the second, what I call for simplicity sake, the economic account, trust depends on the individual abilities of people to trust. These, in turn, depend upon factors such as early childhood experiences and other attributes having to do with the entruster. Thus, trust on this model has to do with certain traits of the entruster, the entrusted, and the context, what the trustee is being trusted with.

Hardin's account is helpful in understanding how some managed-care, cost containment mechanisms can affect trust between doctor and patient. When we consider the fate of trust in the context of aggressively implemented managed care, cost containment mechanisms, its prospects are dim. For example, if trust formation depends upon the entruster's understanding of the interests and incentives of the trustee, then capitated plans will certainly raise questions about physicians' ability to act in the interest of patients, instead of in their own interests. Of course, the public has always viewed members of the healing professions with a measure of ambivalence. In addition, the recent recognition by the Institute of Medicine and others of the numerous medical errors inflicted on patients has only aggravated public suspicion of physicians.[30] Nonetheless, managed care has also had a share in modifying society's picture of the trusting physician—the Marcus Welby that had dominated public perception.

Under the circumstances of compromised trust, patients may lose at least some of the therapeutic benefits associated with a high-trust doctor–patient relationship. I will argue that the fallout from a trust-disabled doctor–patient relationship will extend beyond this particular dyad to the community. Therefore the scope of who and what counts morally in our understanding of the potential costs of managed care, or any health-care system for that matter, needs to be broadened beyond the interests of patients, physicians, and health-care organizations. The doctor–patient relationship should itself be understood as a 'public good.'

By looking at the doctor–patient relationship in a social context, I look at some of the ways that it can potentially benefit the community. This analysis requires looking at the relationship between doctor and patient not solely as a mechanism for the delivery of medical care, but also as a relationship capable of providing its participants with an array of social advantages. A visit to the doctor has the potential to enrich our lives, perhaps by confirming our optimism about the caring qualities of human beings and replenishing our personal reservoir of trust and social capital. Although a number of factors that could be taken into account in attempts to understand the social character of the doctor–patient relationship, I focus on two. In Chapter 4, I consider how the doctor–patient relationship can contribute to health promotion, and how the relationship between doctor and patient may be affected by unequal access to health care.

In Chapter 5, this theme is taken in a different direction when I argue that the doctor–patient relationship has the potential to contribute to our reservoir of social capital. If we view medical care and its provision through insurance as primarily a private matter between individual contractors to be negotiated by them, then to interfere in their relationship, without their consent, would constitute a violation of liberty. Typically, we treat conduct that is primarily private, and can potentially harm no one but the parties involved, with deference and respect. This seems to make good sense in the context of health care because, for the most part, it appears that the brunt of decisions doctors and patients make will be borne by one of the main decision-makers, the patient. Looking at the doctor–patient relationship, not in isolation, but as a part of the social fabric, I pay special attention to the social capital dimension of the medical relationship, noting the important moral implications social capital has for the community. As a significant source of trust, the doctor–patient relationship is also important for social capital. Insofar as managed care undermines trust between doctor and patient, it also risks diminishing our reservoir of social capital.

Chapter 6 shifts the focus of the book from a discussion of the potential moral impact of managed health care on trust and social capital to a discussion of the impact of some of the laws concerning managed care on the reservoir of trust. With the help of the narrative theory of law, I show that some 'legal statements' convey meanings that may discourage the cultivation of trust. I argue that social capital should be among the key canons used in judicial decision-making. This focus continues in Chapter 7, where I look at the role that employers/payers have played in shepherding their employees into managed plans. Here I argue in support of a moral framework that requires greater deference to employee preferences based on both consideration of employers as proxies and concerns about social capital.

Finally, in Chapter 8, I discuss some of the policy implications of this analysis. As we look at what direction health policy should take in the wake of the backlash against managed care, we need to include a consideration of trust and social capital. The harmful consequences of policies that may provide patients with less than explicit information about financial incentives for trust are considered. I also briefly explore the implications for social capital of rationing within a closed or open system, and I discuss an educational approach to reining in health-care costs that has been explored by some employers. Finally, I consider the relevance of strategies used in other social contexts to the health-care context, and the potential of some health-care reform measures used by other nations.

Defining managed care

The term 'managed care' has been defined in a number of ways. Most importantly, managed care combines in one system the functions of insuring or financing care with providing clinical services. Thus, it is a health-care delivery system in which what is delivered is managed by the insurer with the ultimate goal of both providing care and containing costs. I use the term 'managed care' broadly to refer to health plans that use cost containment mechanisms designed to reduce spending on health care by targeting what care is delivered to patients. More specifically, I am interested in those mechanisms that affect physician conduct and the doctor–patient relationship. Although it would be desirable from the perspective of perspicuity to replace the broad usage of the term 'managed care' with a more specific enumeration of containment mechanisms, the term 'managed care' has been used broadly far too long to be dispensed with now. 'Managed care', firmly embedded in everyday usage and is the adopted term of professional and academic journals. Moreover, what makes managed care problematic is not the presence of cost containment mechanisms per se, but the aggressiveness with which the principles of managed care are implemented.

The difficulties inherent in defining 'managed care' are only exacerbated by the fact that the strategies and implementation of managed care are always changing. Still there are some general principles. When care is managed, the insurer plays a more active role than in traditional insurance in determining what is to be done for a patient, where it will be done, who will do it, and what the cost should be. Many of the cost containment mechanisms that managed-care organizations (MCOs) use target physician conduct by shifting the risk of insuring patients from the insurer to the physician. The idea behind this is that if physicians are required to absorb more of the financial risk of care, they will practice more cost-effective care. Although the particular strategies used are constantly changing, the main principles of managed care are relatively stable. For example, managed fee-for-service, a relative new comer to the health-plan landscape, combines fee-for-service payment with payer–provider collaboration on matters such as utilization, and the possible use of incentives for 'high quality and efficient performance.'[31] The use of incentives and utilization review are standard managed-care cost containment strategies.

For the purposes of this book, I am concerned with the aspects of managed care that affect the level of trust between doctor and patient. A number of factors go into determining whether a cost containment strategy will intrude on the relationship between doctor and patient. Susan Dorr Goold points out that whether or not a method of paying physicians adversely affects the doctor–patient relationship depends in part on the amount of money at issue. For example, a capitated system in which physicians are paid a generous per member per month payment in a large group practice is less likely to create adverse conflicts of interest than a parsimonious rate to a solo physician in an urban practice.[32] When a physician has a large number of patients, she can more effectively spread the risk without harming any one patient.[33] Certainly, capitation has great potential to intrude on the trust relationship between doctor and patient. And when per-member amounts are too low they can lead to other problems, such as cherry picking (choosing healthy patients), long waits, and denial of expensive necessary care (referrals). Gate-keeping in tandem with capitation also has the potential to interfere with the quality of the doctor–patient relationship.

But capitation is not the only potentially problematic cost containment mechanism used in managed systems. Salaried mechanisms may also adversely affect trust between doctor and patient. Again, Dorr Goold is instructive. Withholds, for example, amounting to one third of a physician's salary and out of which drugs, referrals, and tests must be paid, can strongly affect physician decision making.[34] Salary combined with a 5–10 percent end-of-the-year bonus, based on factors such as utilization, quality, and patient satisfaction, may have less impact on the doctor–patient relationship, especially if the compensation is high.[35] Whether managed care adversely affects the relationship between doctor and patient depends on a number of factors, most importantly how *aggressively* it is practiced. Thus, it would be a mistake to assume that all managed care will interfere in the relationship between doctor and patient. Even capitation in the right setting and with a generous capitated amount can be relatively benign. Under other circumstances, and with a low per member per month amount, it will lead to harmful intrusions on the doctor–patient relationship. When mechanisms for managing care are implemented, they have the potential to be implemented aggressively and they, in turn, can intrude on the doctor–patient relationship.

The term 'health maintenance organization' (HMO) is often used interchangeably with MCO. Typically, though, HMOs manage care through 'gatekeeper physicians,' primary care physicians who control patient access to services and specialists. As Mashaw and Marmor point out, HMOs achieve savings by eliminating patient self-referral to hospitals and specialists.[36] In contrast, MCOs use other cost-containment mechanisms, such as capitation, shifting the risk of insuring and caring for patients from the insurer to the physician. [37] The extent of the risk assumed by physicians and the degree of pressure they experience will depend largely on the size of the per month capitated amount. Other forms of third-party control of care are 'utilization review,' which involves a formal assessment by the insurer of the appropriateness of the services or treatment plan, and 'clinical practice guideline statements, that guide providers about 'appropriate' care for specific clinical conditions.[38]

Managed care can also be based on a staff model, in which physicians are the salaried employees of an HMO or Group or Network Practice model and contract to provide care to members of the HMO. Indeed, recent manifestations of managed care have included managed fee-for-service, a scheme that blends some of the incentives and utilization tools of managed care with traditional fee-for-service.[39] Finally, notice that the shift from fee-for-service (to managed care involves a shift from retrospective payment to prospective payment and a shift from the provider/patient dyad to the provider/insurer dyad or the patient/provider/insurer triad. Although this broad description of managed care is by no means comprehensive, my purpose has been to give enough background information about managed care to facilitate understanding the moral and social issues raised in this book.

Notes

1 R. Putnam. *Bowling Alone*. New York: Simon & Schuster, 2000, pp. 20–1.
2 J.S. Coleman. Social Capital in the Creation of Human Capital. *American Journal of Sociology,* 1988; 94(suppl): S95–120.
3 R.J. Blendon et al. Understanding the Managed Care Backlash. *Health Affairs,* 17: 1998; 80–94; A.C. Enthoven et al. Consumer Choice and The Managed Care Backlash. *American Journal of Law and Medicine,* 2001; 27: 1–15; H. Taylor. Hostility to Managed Care Continues to Grow; But it is Far from Overwhelming. *Harris Poll #38,* 29 July 1998, online, available HTTP: <http://www.harrisinteractive.com/harris_poll/index.asp?PID=170> (accessed 23 September 2004); J.C. Robinson. The End of Managed Care. *Journal of the American Medical Association,* 2001; 285: 2622–8.
4 More recently, the Supreme Court has weakened its protection of ERISA managed plans, beginning with *Pegram v. Herdrich,* 530 U.S. 211, 120 S.Ct. 2143, 2000, *Rush Prudential HMO v. Moran,* 122 S.Ct. 2151, 2002, *Cicio v. Vytra Health Care,* 321 F.3d 83, 2d Cir 2003, and *Kentucky Association of Health Plans v. Miller,* 123 S. Ct. 1471, 2003.
5 E.H. Morreim. *Balancing Act: The New Medical Ethics of Medicine's New Economics.* Washington, DC: Georgetown University Press, 1995; W. Mariner. Business v. Medical Ethics: Conflicting Standards for Managed Care. *Journal of Law, Medicine and Ethics,* 1995; 23: 241.
6 E. Friedman. Money Isn't Everything: Nonfinancial Barriers to Access. *Journal of the American Medical Association,* 1994; 271: 1535–8; K. Fiscella et al. Inequality in Quality: Addressing Socioeconomic, Racial, and Ethnic Disparities in Health Care. *Journal of the American Medical Association,* 2000; 283: 2579–84.
7 See, for example, M.P. Doescher et al. Racial and Ethnic Disparities in Perceptions of Physician Style and Trust. *Archives of Family Medicine,* 2000; 9: 1156–65.
8 Kaiser Family Foundation. *Chartbook: Trends and Indicators in the Changing Health Care Marketplace.* 2002 Update, Exhibit 2.3.
9 E.H. Morreim. *Holding Health Care Accountable.* New York: Oxford University Press, 2001.
10 J. Gabel et al. Job-Based Health Insurance in 2001: Inflation Hits Double Digits, Managed Care Retreats. *Health Affairs,* 2001; 20: 180.
11 J. Gabel et al. Health Benefits in 2004: Four Years of Double-Digit Premium Increases Take Their Toll On Coverage. *Health Affairs,* 2004; 23: 205.
12 J. Gabel et al. Job-based Benefits in 2002: Some Important Trends. *Health Affairs,* 2002; 21: 143–51. HMO Enrollment on the Decline; PPOs, POS Plans Gain in Membership and Satisfaction Ratings. *Employment Benefit Plan Review,* MA, 2001.
13 G.P. Mays et al. Managed Care Rebound? Recent Changes in Health Plans' Cost Containment Strategies. *Health Affairs,* 11 August 2004, Web Exclusive W4, pp. 427–36.
14 M.K. Wynia et al. Physician Manipulation of Reimbursement Rules for Patients: Between a Rock and a Hard Place. *Journal of the American Medical Association,* 2000; 238: 1861.

15 E.J. Emanuel and N. Neveloff Dubler. Preserving the Physician–Patient Relationship in the Era of Managed Care. *Journal of the American Medical Association*, 1995; 273: 323–9.

16 Mariner, op. cit., pp. 240–1.

17 *Canterbury v. Spence*, U.S. Court of Appeals, District of Columbia Circuit, 19 May 1972, 464 Federal Reporter, 2nd Series 772.

18 J.S. House et al. Social Relationships and Health. In I. Kawachi et al. (eds). *The Society and Population Health Reader: Income Inequality and Health*. Vol. 1. New York: New Press, 1999, pp. 161–70; L.F. Berkman. The Role of Social Relations in Health Promotion. In Kawachi et al., op. cit., pp. 171–83.

19 House et al., op. cit.; I. Kawachi et al. Social Capital, Income Inequality and Mortality. In Kawachi et al., op. cit., pp. 222–35.

20 A.K. Shapiro. Patient–Provider Relationships and the Placebo Effect. In *Behavior Health*. New York: J. Wiley and Sons, 1984, p. 3781; S.H. Kaplan et al. Assessing the Effects of Physician–Patient Interaction on the Outcomes of Chronic Disease. *Medical Care*, 1989; 27: S5110–27.

21 R. Kuttner. The American Health Care System: Employer-Sponsored Health Coverage. *New England Journal of Medicine*, 1999; 340: 248–52.

22 The Health of Nations: A Survey of Health-Care Finance. *The Economist*, 17 July 2004, p. 5.

23 Ibid.

24 R. Short, Chairman. Griffiths NHS Management Inquiry Report. *House of Commons, Social Services Committee*, 20 June 1984. See also: M.L. Lassey et al. *Health Care Systems Around the World*. Upper Saddle River, NJ: Prentice Hall Press, 1997, p. 223.

25 Lassey et al., op. cit., p. 329.

26 S. Stevens. Reform Strategies for the English NHS. *Health Affairs*, 2004; 23: 40.

27 Ibid.

28 Lassey et al., op. cit., p. 91.

29 A.C. Kao et al. The Relationship Between Method of Physician Payment and Patient Trust. *Journal of the American Medical Association*, 1998; 280: 1708–14; D. Mechanic and M. Schlesinger. The Impact of Managed Care on Patients' Trust in Medical Care and Their Physicians. *Journal of the American Medical Association*, 1996; 275: 1693–7.

30 The Institute of Medicine. *To Err is Human: Building a Safer Health System*. Washington, DC: The National Academies, 1999; L. Leape. Error in Medicine. *Journal of the American Medical Association*, 1994; 272: 1851–7.

31 University of Maryland Center on Aging. *Applying Managed Fee-for-Service Delivery Models to Improve Care for Dually Eligible Beneficiaries*. MMIP Technical Assistance Paper No. 12, University of Southern Maine, 2002, p. 3.

32 S. Dorr Good. Money and Trust: Relationships between Patients, Physicians, and Health Plans. *Journal of Health Politics, Policy and Law*, 1998; 23: 690.

33 Ibid.

34 Ibid., p. 691.

35 Ibid.

36 J.L. Mashaw and T.R. Marmor. Conceptualizing, Estimating and Reforming Fraud, Waste, and Abuse in Healthcare Spending. *Yale Journal on Regulation*, 1994; 11: 490.

37 American Medical Association. *Managing Managed Care in the Medical Practice*. Norcross, GA: Coker Publishing, 1996, p. 14.

38 Ibid., p. 15.

39 See, for example, S.S. Wallack and C.P. Tompkins, Realigning Incentives in Fee-for-Service Medicare; A Proposal to Reform Medicare Payment while Retaining the Fee-for-Service System. *Health Affairs*, 2003; 22: 59–70.

1 Conflicting values in a troubled health-care system

Surveys, studies, and polls tell a story of public concern with managed care.[1] Since 1997, there has been a 22 percent decline in the proportion of the public that says that managed care is doing a good job.[2] Moreover, in the years 1995–2000, the number of Americans who believed that the growth of managed care is 'a bad thing' grew from 28 percent to 52 percent.[3] And many Americans believe that managed care has the potential to harm the quality of medical care.[4] Whether those surveyed base their opinion on good information or even understand their own health plans is another matter.[5]

Patients and other 'consumers' of health care are not the only ones concerned with medicine under managed care. Some of those working within the medical system, such as medical students, residents, faculty, and deans, view managed care in negative terms.[6] In a comprehensive survey Simon et al. found that a majority of these medical professionals rated fee-for-service better than managed care with respect to access to care, minimizing ethical conflicts and the quality of the doctor–patient relationship.[7] Although other studies indicate that there are no clear quality differences between managed care and fee-for-service, many people remain dissatisfied with managed care.[8] In recent years, there has been a 'backlash' against managed care, followed by a decline in enrollment in strictly managed plans,[9] and then a reintroduction of once-abandoned cost containment strategies.[10] There has also been a recent spate of state mandates enacted to remedy some of the perceived problems with managed care,[11] and the federal Patients' Bill of Rights awaits congressional action. Indeed, until recently, there was some indication that the Supreme Court may be enhancing protection for patients in managed-care plans, as the cases of *Pegram v. Herdrich*,[12] *Rush Prudential v. Moran*,[13] and *Kentucky Association of Health Plans, Inc. v. Miller* seem to indicate.[14] However, the Court may be backtracking on this 'trend' in *Aetna Health, Inc. v. Davila*, when it decided that an HMO's refusal to provide physician-recommended medical care, resulting in harm to the patient, was subject to federal preemption.[15]

Patient health is, of course, among the main purposes of medicine. But medicine is also a social institution that contributes to the community. Thus changes in how health care is delivered have the potential to affect not only those who receive care, but the community in which they live. It would be a mistake to ignore the impact of the health-care system on the community. In view of how much trust patients have traditionally had for their physicians, and the connection between trust and social capital, the doctor–patient relationship is likely an important source of social capital.

The cost of care

Managed medical care was adopted as a way to control escalating health-care costs. In the United States, health care is expensive. In 2002, national health spending increased to $1.6 trillion, and health spending's share of the GDP rose to 14.9 percent, the largest annual increases in each case since 1993.[16] The Health Care Finance Administration (HCFA) projected that, by 2012, national health expenditures will total 3.1 trillion, an estimated 17.7 percent of the GDP.[17]

Other Western countries spend much less on health care, and many of them provide some version of universal access to health care. In 2002, France spent 9.7 percent of its GDP on health care, Britain 7.7 percent, and Canada 9.6 percent. During the same year, the U.S. spent 14.6 percent of its GDP on health care.[18] Although the U.S. spends a greater percentage of its GDP on health care, 45 million Americans were without health insurance in 2003—15 percent of the population.[19] Moreover, although the U.S. spends more on health care than other Western countries, Americans by no means have the best health status. When compared with other member countries of the Organization for Economic Co-Operation and Development (OECD) on standard health status measures, the U.S. compares poorly. In 1998, female life expectancy at birth was 81.4 in Canada, 81.6 in Italy, and 84 in Japan. It was 79.4 in the U.S.[20] Male life expectancy was 75.8 in Canada, 75.3 in Italy, 77.2 in Japan, and 73.9 in the U.S.[21] Although life expectancy at birth is only one measure of health status, the U.S. compares poorly with other countries on a number of health status measures, including life expectancy at 65, infant mortality, and premature mortality.[22] Health expenditures are not the only factor to contribute to health status; still, these results are surprising given the amount of money the U.S. spends on health care.

It is paradoxical, to say the least, that the U.S. spends as much money on health care as it does and yet experiences extensive dissatisfaction with the product.[23] Although a number of explanations have been given to explain the high cost of medical care in the United States, and the matter is complex, there are two views that stand out. The first claims that health insurance under fee-for-service gives neither patients nor providers an incentive to use resources efficiently. According to this view, both patients and their doctors spend recklessly on health care, with no appreciation for what health services may cost. This explanation does not, however, explain the recent increase in health-care costs under managed care. In the second view, the high cost of health care is attributed to the consumption of high-tech medicine—especially by the elderly.[24] Any effort to slow the ever-rising cost of health expenditures must address the consumption of health care by a small, but high-cost population, including the elderly and the dying.[25] Still others explain the difference between the U.S. and other OECD countries on higher prices in the U.S. for health-care services and goods.[26]

Spending on health care occurs in both public and private spheres. Government spending at the federal, state, and local levels rose in 2000 to $587.2 billion,[27] or 45 percent of the total,[28] an increase from 41 percent in 1990.[29] In 2002, public spending accounted for about 46 percent of all national health-care spending while the rest was spent privately.[30] Employers and employees are the most significant spenders in the sphere of private, health-care spending. Private spending increased significantly in 2002, up from 6.7 percent in 2000 to 9.3 percent.[31] The number of people in the U.S. population covered by employment-based health insurance went down in 2003 from 61.3 percent to 60.4 percent, while the number of people covered by government health insurance rose, from 25.7 percent to 26.6 percent. (The rise in government spending is likely due to an increase in the number of people covered by Medicaid.)[32] Because employers are responsible for such a large portion of health-care spending, they have a strong incentive to find a cost effective approach to insuring their employees.[33] As we shall see in Chapter 7, employers have considerable influence on the nature and quality of health care in the U.S.

Beginning in 1992, earlier growth in health-care spending temporarily stabilized, primarily because of the cost containment efforts of managed care.[34] Some have argued that managed care achieved these slower rates by slowing down the rate at which new and expensive technologies are diffused.[35] Others have speculated that the rise in health-care costs has slowed because of the recent decline in the number of insured people.[36] According to the latter, when individuals have health insurance, they seek out health services since they either will not have to pay for the individual services or will only have to pay a fraction of the cost.[37] Although the matter is complex, it can be recast in more benign terms. We might say, for example, that health insurance gives people the freedom to seek medical care when they are sick or worried about their health. The uninsured will be discouraged from turning to the health-care system when they are ill or concerned about their health.[38] In any case, it is likely that as the number of uninsured increases as it has in the recent past, we can anticipate a restraining influence on expenditures.[39]

If we consider that (1) the U.S. can look forward to spending 18.4 percent of its GDP on health care by the year 2013,[40] and that (2) the amount spent on health care by the U.S. has been substantially larger than that spent by any other country for decades,[41] these facts suggest the need to engage in some kind of rationing of health care. However, (1) and (2) do not tell us what to ration, how much to ration, or how to ration. Americans value their health and the activities that good health permits. Commenting on our bleak history with health-care cost containment, Drew Altman and Larry Levitt state that it may be impossible to control spending on health for any length of time. They speculate that the American appetite for the latest and the best health care may be responsible for high expectations.[42] Wendy Mariner has argued that the call for health-care rationing lacks real credibility to the American population because the claim of scarcity is somewhat artificial.[43]

When we talk about the need to ration health care and what counts as excessive spending on health care, it is important to keep in mind that health care represents one seventh of the U.S. economy and, in turn, that a number of economic interests and agendas are invested in the health-care industry.[44] We need to be mindful that lowering the costs of health care will lower costs for some and perhaps increase costs for others; and while some costs may be decreased, the profits of others may still be increased. For example, stemming the rise of expenditures on health care during the mid 1990s allowed insurance companies to increase their profits.[45] The relativity of our evaluations of health-care costs is nicely stated by Chernew; 'a portion of rising health-care costs may simply be a transfer from consumers of health care to suppliers without a net loss in aggregate welfare.' Chernew also states that 'health-care cost growth is not necessarily undesirable if consumers are willing to pay for the costs associated with new technology.'[46]

The view that managed care will reduce the use of expensive medical technology should also be looked at carefully.[47] The Health Care Financing Administration (HCFA) speculates that growth in health-care expenditures will resume. Those who believe that the decline in expenditures of the 1990s was based on the transition from fee-for-service to managed care also believe that the decline will be short-term. If lower expenditures are due to a slower diffusion of technology, some health economists challenge the ability of managed care to contain these costs over time.[48] Thus, it is far from obvious that once we grant the need to ration health care, managed care will be the optimal mechanism to effectively curb the growth of health-care expenditures.[49]

Because physicians affect so much of health-care spending, cost containment mechanisms that target physician behavior and, in turn, the doctor–patient relationship, have been widely implemented by managed-care plans as a way to rein in escalating medical expenditures. This, in turn, I think, has affected trust between doctor and patient. I shall argue that trust and social capital should not be negotiated in the hope of lowering health-care costs. They are far too important to our health and to the welfare of the community. Finally, keep in mind that money that is saved on the health care of one patient will not necessarily be spent on the health care of another patient or on some other morally worthy causes.[50] Instead, in for-profit plans, these 'savings' may well be reflected in the salaries of Chief

Executive Officers (CEOs), the profits of shareholders of MCOs, or payers. In any case, since health-care spending is again on the upswing, it is clear neither that managed care has fulfilled its promise to increase access to health care by making it more affordable nor that it can.[51]

Ethical assumptions, principles and theories

A number of different ethical concepts surface in this book. In general, my analysis is based on consequentialism, the view that morally right actions are to be identified by the good outcomes that they bring.[52] Informed by this ethical approach, I have reframed questions about the impact of managed care on the doctor–patient relationship to questions about the effect of the current health-care system the community at large. From a consequentialist perspective, there is no good reason to restrict our analysis of the consequences of an organization's actions on its immediate constituents. The main concern of a consequentalist approach is with the impact of those organizations on the community. By shifting the scope of the analysis from patient and organizational welfare to community welfare and from patient 'rights' to community 'rights,' I am, in turn, identifying new criteria for evaluating both health plans and the doctor–patient relationship permitted by them. Of course, the welfare of individual patients still counts, but so does the community in which they live. Similarly, health outcomes are important, but so are the levels of satisfaction that patients and the community experience with the health-care system. It does not, however, follow that because I am looking at the consequences of managed care for society care that I do not also look at the costs and benefits to patients—the immediate recipients of health care. Trust and social capital promote good health outcomes for patients and community alike.[53] However, my analysis is, at the same time, limited. I do not take into account *all* of the considerations that would be required for a complete analysis of the issues at hand.

Many of the ethical problems raised in this book will also be considered through the lens of the professional ethics of fiduciaries. The concept of a 'fiduciary' may be understood narrowly to refer to a specific set of legal duties, or broadly to include the professional ethics of fiduciaries. Because physicians' conduct suggests that they have assumed more extensive professional obligations than are dictated by, for example, the American Medical Association (AMA) Code of Ethics,[54] this broader definition is particularly appropriate. Although the concept of a 'fiduciary' duty may seem inconsistent with consequentialism, traditional fiduciary ethics can be justified on consequentialist grounds.[55] That is, fiduciary duties can take the place of more expensive and possibly less efficient mechanisms for protecting vulnerable clients. Paradoxically, some of the ethical problems that are associated with managed care are driven by the fiduciary ethics of corporations, in an ethic similar to professional medical ethics.[56] For example, cost containment mechanisms that limit a physician's autonomy (utilization review) can qualify as morally problematic from the perspective of the fiduciary ethics of physicians and are at the same time motivated by the fiduciary duties of management to their shareholders.

Fiduciary law is based on the law of trusts.[57] In the trust relationship one person holds the property of another for the benefit of the beneficiary.[58] In paradigmatic fiduciary relationships such as this one, it is difficult for the beneficiary to monitor what the trustee does. In part because of this, fiduciaries are typically under special duties to avoid self-dealing and conflicts of interest. Where there is a significant power imbalance, as in the relationship between trustee and beneficiary, the higher duties of fiduciaries may be invoked. Thus fiduciary duties are often imputed to professionals.

In law, doctors have specific, as opposed to global, fiduciary duties to patients. Unlike, for example, the directors of a corporation, who have 'an open-ended duty to maximize the beneficiaries' wealth,' under the law physicians have narrowly defined fiduciary duties with respect to certain specific tasks. Fiduciary law has been applied to physicians with respect to (1) the duty not to abandon patients, (2) the duty to maintain confidences, and (3) the duty to obtain informed consent to treatment.[59] In addition, although the courts have vacillated on this, in *Moore v. Regent of the University of California* it was recognized that connected with the fiduciary duty to obtain informed consent is (4) a duty to disclose any personal interest unrelated to the patient's health, such as research and economic interests that may affect a doctor's judgment.[60] And in *Wickline v. State of California*, although there is some confusion about the court's holding, it was indicated that, given a physician's fiduciary duty to patients and the prevailing standard of practice, physicians may have a duty to advocate for patients when payers deny medically necessary care.[61]

There are fiduciary-based objections to managed care stemming from issues surrounding the disclosure of information to patients. Patients who enroll in managed-care plans, often through their employment, may not have full information about the benefits in the plan prior to enrolling. It is also unclear just what the duties of health plans and physicians are with respect to disclosing the nature of financial incentives. But even when subscribers are provided with documentation of the terms of the plans, they may not understand the meaning of such terms.[62] They may not know, for instance, that 'medical necessity' is a term of exclusion.[63] The gag clauses once included in some managed-care contracts prevented physicians from disclosing some information to patients.[64] Gag clauses not only had the potential to interfere with informed consent, but they also compromised a doctor's fiduciary duty to patients.[65]

Some of the perceived problems that have been associated with managed care with respect to patients and physicians can partially be explained by the moral strength of managed care with respect to its own shareholders. In the case of for-profit MCOs, containing costs and, in turn, increasing profits for their shareholders are based on the fiduciary duty of care to shareholders and the moral presuppositions that underlie it.[66] As the agents of shareholders, managers are under a duty to maximize the interests of stockholders.[67] It is not just that business is interested in making a profit; instead, it is that the ethics of business is that managers and directors are morally obligated to act in the interest of shareholders. Whether or not this view of corporate duties exaggerates the interest in profit maximization, clearly, cost containment figures importantly in managed-care medicine, both from the perspective of health-care organizations and the employers who pay them. Moreover, as is often the case, managers are also shareholders and may receive compensation in stock options. These methods of compensation only combine with the duty of care to enhance the commitment of managers to the bottom line.

The ethics of contract explains another, although more limited, set of ethical problems that have surfaced in discussions about managed care. In one widely used definition of 'contract,' 'a contract is a promise enforceable at law.'[68] According to *Black's Law Dictionary*, [its] essentials are competent parties, subject matter, a legal consideration, mutuality of agreement, and mutuality of obligations.'[69] Contracts express our legal system's commitment to the idea that people's freely chosen agreements should be respected.

Some of the web of relationships that comprise managed care are contract based.[70] According to contract principles, the rights and obligations of the parties are specified in the contract. In the absence of a contract, there are no legal rights except as specified by law. Doctor and MCO, MCO and employer, and MCO and subscriber have relationships based on contract and out of these contracts come specific rights and obligations. In general, the law defers to the contracts made by people under fair conditions of bargaining. The ethic inherent in contract is parallel to the ethics of respect for the autonomous and consensual arrangements of individuals.[71]

According to contract principles, subscribers are entitled only to those benefits that have been specified in the contract. For those who endorse a contract-based ethic, the objection that MCOs are morally problematic because they deny patients beneficial medical care would only be persuasive if managed care were in breach of contract—if, having promised a certain level of care, MCOs failed to provide it. The ethics of contract cannot explain why it is morally problematic for MCOs to deny beneficial care when patients consent to that denial of care, unless of course, the quality of consent is challenged. In this way, the obligations of care specified by a contract can be very different, for example, from those that would be generated by the American Medical Association's requirement that physicians provide materially beneficial care and the common law as seen in *Wickline*. Arguably, when a physician's professional and fiduciary duties are taken into account, it is difficult not to conclude that there is a duty of advocacy of medically beneficial care, regardless of contractual consent to less-than-beneficial care.

Stewardship, social justice and contributive justice

Discussions about the ethics of managed care have also involved appeals to the ethics of stewardship, social justice, and contributive justice. Although I do not use these concepts in this book, they have been invoked to justify rationing by MCOs and, in turn, physician departures from fiduciary duties. Some familiarity with them is therefore necessary as background.

MCOs are both insurers and providers of care. In their capacity as insurers, they have obligations to all plan members to provide contracted-for benefits—usually 'medically necessary' care. James Sabin, in an essay devoted to defending the duty of physicians to engage in bedside rationing, states that at present 'Insurers take care of stewardship,' which he defines as 'seeking fairness for the population.'[72] Moreover, although not stated, Sabin appears to believe that the obligations of stewardship that he attributes to insurers and which he believes physicians ought to assume are over society's resources.[73] Insurers are viewed as denying benefits to some patients in order to provide them to other needy and deserving patients. Moreover, although this is less clear, Sabin seems to believe that the resources at issue belong to society and have been 'given' to insurers for just this purpose—they are the stewards of treasured social resources. Thus insurers who permit individual patients to consume more than their fair share of these medical resources have committed an injustice against both the other patients to whom they have obligations and the community that entrusted them with these resources.

Nancy Jecker gives an explanation for some of the thinking that may lie behind support for the duty of stewardship:[74]

> Medicine comprises a social institution responsible not only for the care of individual sick people, but also for distributing the benefits and burdens of social life. Professional accountability is not exclusive to the patient, but to the society that the institution of medicine served. As a consequence, the ethics of the medical profession cannot be adequately understood in a vacuum. While fidelity to one's patients and to the bond between patient and physician is important, it is not an ethical absolute. Instead, fidelity must be considered in tandem with other important values, such as social justice.

Although Jecker is addressing the more complicated case of physicians, presumably some of the same considerations would apply to insurers, especially insurers that are also involved in providing care. Moreover, if Jecker's analysis of the fidelity between doctor and patient is right and if, as she believes, physicians err too much on the side of patient loyalty, then the case for insurers should be that much easier to make since they may not be fettered by the same fiduciary duties to individual patients as physicians.

Insurers have obligations to all of those plan members with whom they have contracted. But it is not clear that they have these obligations in virtue of a social contract with the community. Nor is it clear in what sense the resources 'belong' to society. MCOs, in their capacity as insurers, do of course have obligations to a number of insured, not simply to one patient. Of course, they also have contractual obligations to individuals. These obligations are derived from contractual agreements between patients and insurers. Although the obligations themselves will vary from contract to contract, typically they include an obligation to provide 'medically necessary' health-care benefits. Unfortunately, what will qualify as medically necessary care is notoriously unclear, as is the question of *who* is permitted to determine medical necessity: patients, physicians, the MCO itself, or a third party (external review/second opinion). The Supreme Court has recently addressed this question in *Rush Prudential v. Moran*.[75] Sometimes the definition of 'medical necessity' will be provided by the MCO in the contract, though this does not ensure perspicuity of meaning. Haavi Morriem has coined the term 'contributive justice' to explain the idea that there are duties to provide care to all of those who have contributed to the 'pot.'[76]

Even if MCOs are not the stewards of social resources, they clearly have contractually specific obligations to *all* plan members. If MCOs permit any single patient to receive care in excess of those contractual obligations, and they do so at the peril of other plan members, then they have wronged them. But this wrong would seem to be in the nature of a breach of contract or, in the language of ethics, a broken promise or a failure to respect autonomy.

The idea that rationing within a managed system can be justified on the grounds of social justice is in my view mistaken. It assumes a closed system in which resources are moved within the system among needy patients. But is this model widespread? Insofar as this is an accurate picture of managed care, it would be so with respect to not-for-profit managed care in which 91 to 93 percent of the premium dollar goes back into health-care services.[77] However, the trend in HMO enrollment is in the direction of for-profit HMOs, with most Americans who are enrolled in HMOs, enrolled in for-profit, shareholder-owned plans.[78] Since 63.5 percent of people enrolled in HMOs receive their care in for-profit organizations, money not spent on one patient's care might well be spent on administrative costs, paying dividends to shareholders, or paying off the golden parachutes for CEOs.[79] In any case, for-profits attempt to return only 70–80 percent of premiums to health-care services. The rest is divided between shareholders (10–12 percent) and administrative costs.[80] In view of this, it is a fiction to describe the distribution of resources within managed care as based on a social justice ethic. Framing it in this way fails to take into account the implications of for-profit health-care organizations and the orientation of such organizations to their shareholders.[81] Under these circumstances, the question is whether physicians should cooperate with decisions to deny beneficial care, knowing that such care could be provided were more funds devoted to health care.

Certainly some of the earlier HMOs, such as Kaiser Permanente, reflected a social justice ethic.[82] But these are not the same plans as those with which we live today. In Wendy Mariner's description of the problems that confront efforts to ration care in this country, she points out that health-care expenditures are made on the basis of the private decisions of private health insurers, self-insured employers, and individual patients. This has two important implications. First, she points out that there is 'no pre-imposed natural limit on how much money will be spent on health care' and second, from the perspective of patients, health-care resources may appear unlimited.[83] According to Mariner,[84]

> If the amount of money allocated to health care is substantially deter-mined by private market decisions, there does not appear to be any jus-tification for rationing. After all, the amount of money in any single health care pot can be increased or decreased at any time. Thus, the health care resources available to patients are not fixed and scarce but can be increased or decreased. In a market system, limits on the amount of money spent for health care can be or appear arbitrary or unfair.

The distinction that Mariner wants to make is one between artificially imposed limits such as those that characterize a market system of health care and the naturally imposed limits on a resource, such as organs. 'Today's ad hoc limits on the amount of money in the multitude of health care pots do not create credible scarcity.'[85] Arguments supporting the conclusion that insurers must limit care to plan members and must place burdens on the doctor–patient relationship because of justice-based consid-erations to other plan members are weak. Rationing based on artificially imposed limits does not command the same moral authority that can be marshaled with a genuine scarcity of resources or can be justified on the basis of good moral reasons. Yes MCOs have obligations to all of their members, but in specific cases of withholding beneficial care, matters are complex and a number of questions can be raised.[86]

Many health plans, of course, also have obligations to shareholders, payers/employers, and administrators. The question can always be asked, 'Why can't more money be put in the "pot"?' And from an ethics perspec-tive, it is always right to ask what criteria are used to determine how much money to put in the 'pot.' Did the 'pot' contain an adequate amount to meet contractual obligations in the first place? Was the contract fair or unfair? Was it conscionable or unconscionable? Was there, in fact, a meeting of the minds? And of course, we can always challenge the ethical paradigm under-lying the contract on the basis of substantive principles of distribution, such as utilitarian ones. There is some evidence from the study undertaken by Wynia et al. that physicians would be more willing to help health plans save money if they knew that the benefit saved would be conferred on other patients.[87] In Chapter 7, I argue that the principles that ought to guide employers involved in plan design are standards of 'rationality, fairness, and effectiveness' and that a bottom-up approach that honors the professional ethics of physicians should be reflected.

There are other reasons why the social justice perspective may not work as applied to physicians in for-profit health plans. As hybrids, MCOs combine the functions of insuring and providing care. Toward meeting the second function, they use the services of physicians and other providers, sometimes requiring them to rein in some of their patient advocacy duties in the service of their social justice duties.[88] There has been a great deal written about whether or not physicians in managed plans act ethically when they withhold beneficial care from patients. Jecker and others have argued that physicians within an MCO who fall short of advocacy for their patients, and who thereby appear to compromise their professional obligations, nonetheless meet their 'broader social responsibilities.'[89] In addition to being unclear legally,[90] this argument seems weak as a moral argument when applied to for-profit health plans. Here one would have to show that, at least in some cases, sacrificing patient welfare for the sake of shareholder welfare was in the social interest. Harry Nelson, in a report of the Milbank Memorial Fund, seems to echo this view of the corporation when he says, 'Investor-owned HMOs contribute to the public good by increasing the value of shareholders' equity, which in turn benefits the economy.'[91]

But this is not the argument defended by Jecker and those who support the duty of stewardship. One could also argue that a physician's duty of 'zealous advocacy' is a form of role differentiation, an exemption given to physicians from standard moral principles or duties.[92] If, in turn, this exemption were to be lifted, then physicians would be free to act on general moral principles of social justice. Nancy Jecker makes this case. She claims that much advocacy can be sacrificed without cost, for example, to trust within the doctor–patient relationship.[93] Fidelity to patients is a complex matter that no doubt has social, legal, moral, and psychological ramifications. To evaluate the consequences of nibbling away at the duty is similarly complex and requires a comprehensive consideration of the various functions served by the duty.

As I mentioned earlier in this chapter, duties of fidelity are often invoked in relationships where there is an imbalance of power.[94] In these cases, they can act as a substitute for the monitoring mechanisms that might otherwise oversee the conduct of the person who holds power. In view of the vulnerability of patients, because they are sick and fragile, and also because of a difference in expertise between patient and physician, the duty of fidelity serves as a substitute for the inability of patients to properly and effectively monitor the performance of their physicians.[95]

Fidelity to patients might also serve as a psychological mechanism to help physicians monitor their own conduct vis-à-vis patients, a potentially weaker party easily exploited by opportunistic physicians. Physicians who are able to remind themselves on a regular and frequent basis that they are obligated to act in the patient's interest may find that such reminders help them to effectively avoid temptation to self-deal at the patient's expense. Physicians are often as willing as the next person to act selfishly. By diluting duties of fidelity and fostering physician discretion to choose when to serve patient interests and when not to, we may indirectly encourage opportunistic behavior by physicians. This point is made by Simon Ellis in a letter to the editor that appeared in the *British Medical Journal*. He wrote, 'Once one departs from the aim of providing the best possible care for the patient in front of you, it is too easy to be influenced by prejudice . . . making the clinician responsible for rationing puts too much power in one person's hands.'[96] When the patient becomes just one among many interested parties in the 'social institute' that comes to constitute health care, the potential for physician self-dealing may increase.

The view that MCOs and their physician 'agents' are justified in diluting their professional duties to particular patients on the basis of social justice considerations seems most plausible when we ground it on a fictionalized view of managed care, according to which only needy patients will benefit from our sacrifices. But in today's complex medical world this is not the case. To sum up, I have argued that the social justice approach to understanding the ethics of MCOs is problematic because (1) it appears to conflate duties based on contract or agreement with duties based on principles of justice, (2) it seems to misunderstand the self-interested nature of the vying constituencies (in the case of for-profit HMOs) and the role that fidelity plays in protecting patients, and (3) it ignores the moral significance of rationing within an open system.

The social justice argument also assumes that were it not for duties of fidelity to patients, physicians would be free to act on principles of social justice. But surely, in the absence of a special duty, we are not all obligated by justice to serve the interests of all. At this time, duties of social justice are at best supererogatory. It would take an independent argument to show that physicians free of duties of fidelity now have duties of social justice. Perhaps the view is that physicians who serve all plan members *de facto* serve social justice. But this is not persuasive. It is certainly not persuasive in the case of the for-profit plans which constitute most of the plans in which Americans are enrolled. Similarly, physicians who leave one 'ordinary plan' to join a luxury or boutique practice, can serve all the members within their practice, but many people would be hard-pressed to call this meeting their obligations of social justice. In contrast, it is much easier to view physicians who provide free care in developing countries as acting on an ethic of social justice. In the end, it does matter morally where the money is going and why it is not going to what seems to be a morally worthwhile cause. There is more to the story than mere contributive justice.

My argument does not appeal to considerations of social justice. Instead,

I use the concepts of consequentialism and social capital. Nonetheless, I have briefly explained why I believe that appeals to stewardship, social justice, and contributive justice are inadequate as explanations for the rationing-based intrusions on the doctor–patient relationship. When thinking about the obligations of organizations and physicians, it is difficult to understand what all of the moral fuss is about if we do not understand that medicine and business are both guided by fiduciary duties, duties that in this instance conflict with each other.

Notes

1 For a review and analysis of the so-called 'backlash against managed care,' see R.J. Blendon et al. Understanding the Managed Care Backlash. *Health Affairs*, 1998; 17: 80–94; A. Enthoven and S. Singer. The Managed Care Backlash and the Task Force in California. *Health Affairs*, 1998; 17: 95–110; T. Bodenheimer. The HMO Backlash—Righteous or Reactionary? *New England Journal of Medicine*, 1996; 335: 1601–4.

2 R.J. Blendon and J.M. Benson. Americans' Views on Health Policy: A Fifty-Year Historical Perspective. *Health Affairs*, 2001; 20: 40; see also R.H. Miller and H.S. Luft. Does Managed Care Lead to Better or Worse Quality of Care? *Health Affairs*, 1997; 16: 7–25.

3 H. Taylor. Hostility to Managed Care Continues to Grow, But It Is Far From Overwhelming. *Harris Poll #38*, 29 July 1998, available at <http://www.harris interactive.com/harris_poll/index.asp?PID=170> (accessed 23 September 2004).

4 Ibid.

5 P.J. Cunningham et al. Do Consumers Know How Their Health Plan Works. *Health Affairs*, 2001; 20: 159–66, suggesting that fewer than one third of consumers understand the main features of their plans, and in general they tend to over-report restrictions; see also S.L. Isaacs. Consumers' Information Needs: Results of a National Survey. *Health Affairs*, 1996; 15: 31–41.

6 S.R. Simon et al. Views of Managed Care—A Survey of Students, Residents, Faculty and Deans at Medical Schools in the United States. *New England Journal of Medicine*, 1999; 340: 930.

7 Ibid.

8 For a good review of the literature, see R. Adams Dudley et al. The Impact of Financial Incentives on Quality of Health Care. *Milbank Quarterly*, 1998; 76: 649–86; Miller and Luft, op. cit.

9 Kaiser Family Foundation. *Chartbook: Trends and Indicators in the Changing Health Care Marketplace*, May 2002, p. 20.

10 G.P. Mays et al. Managed Care Rebound? Recent Changes in Health Plans' Cost Containment Strategies. *Health Affairs*, 11 August 2004, Web Exclusive W4, pp. 427–36.

11 G. Jenson and M. Morrisey. Employer-Sponsored Health Insurance and Mandated Benefit Laws. *Milbank Quarterly*, 1999; 77: 425–59.

12 *Pegram v. Herdrich*, 530 US 211, 120 S.Ct. 2143, 2000.

13 *Rush Prudential HMO, Inc. v. Moran*, 122 S.Ct. 2151, 2002.

14 *Kentucky Association of Health Plans, Inc. v. Miller*, 123 S. Ct. 1471, 2003.

15 *Aetna Health, Inc. v. Davila*, 124 S. Ct. 2488, 2004.

16 K. Levit et al. Inflation Spurs Health Spending in 2000. *Health Affairs*, 2002; 21: 172; K. Levit et al. Health Spending Rebound Continues in 2002. *Health Affairs*, 2004; 23: 147.

17 S. Heffler et al. Health Spending Projections for 2002–2012. *Health Affairs*, 7 January 2003, Web Exclusive W3, p. 54.

18 OECD, *Table 10: Total expenditure on health, %GDP*. OECD Health Data 2004—Frequently Requested Data, 3 June 2004. Online, available HTTP: <http://www.oecd.org> (accessed 15 September 2004).

19 C. DeNavas-Walt et al. Income, Poverty, and Health Insurance Coverage in the United States: 2003. *Current Population Reports* of U.S. Census Bureau Department of Commerce Economics, and Statistics Administration, August 2004, p. 14.

20 OECD, *Table 1: Life expectancy (in years)*. OECD Health Data 2004—Frequently Requested Data, 3 June 2004. Available at <http://www.oecd.org> (accessed 15 September 2004).

21 Ibid.

22 Ibid.

23 For a recent study of consumer experiences, see Kaiser Family Foundation/ Harvard School of Public Health. National Survey of Consumer Experiences with and Attitudes Toward Health Plans, August 2001; *Harris Poll*, 12–16 December 2003, as described in Many Happy with Health Insurance, Harris Poll Shows. *Heath Care Strategic Management*, 2003; 21: 15.

24 M.L. Berk and A.C. Monheit. The Concentration of Health Care Expenditures, Revisited. *Health Affairs*, 2001; 20: 10.

25 Ibid., pp. 9–18.

26 G.F. Anderson et al. It's the Prices, Stupid: Why The United States Is So Different From Other Countries. *Health Affairs*, 2003; 22: 103.

27 K. Levit et al. Inflation Spurs Health Spending in 2000. *Health Affairs*, 2002; 21: 176.

28 Levit, op. cit., p. 172.

29 K. Levit et al. Trends In U.S. Health Care Spending, 2001. *Health Affairs*, 2003; 22: 162.

30 K. Levit et al. Health Spending Rebound Continues in 2002. *Health Affairs*, 2004; 23: 151.

31 Ibid.

32 DeNavas-Walt et al., op. cit., p. 14.

33 J.K. Iglehart. Changing Health Insurance Trends. *New England Journal of Medicine*, 2002; 347: 957.

34 J.K. Iglehart. The American Health Care System—Expenditures. *New England Journal of Medicine*, 1999; 340: 70–6.

35 M. Chernew et al. Managed Care, Medical Technology, and Health Care Cost Growth: A Review of the Evidence. *Medical Care Research and Review*, 1998; 55: 259–97.

36 S. Smith et al. The Next Ten Years of Health Spending: What Does the Future Hold? *Health Affairs*, 1998; 17: 133.

37 Ibid.

38 For more on the costs of health care as a limit to patients obtaining care, see R.J. Blendon et al. Inequities in Health Care: A Five-Country Survey. *Health Affairs*, 2002; 21: 182–91.

39 Smith, op. cit.

40 S. Heffler et al. Health Spending Projections Through 2013. *Health Affairs*, 11 February 2004, Web Exclusive W4, p. 79.

41 OECD, op. cit., *Table 10: Total expenditure on health, %GDP*.

42 D. Altman and L. Levitt. The Sad History of Health Care Cost Containment as Told in One Chart. *Health Affairs*, 23 January 2002, Web exclusive W83, p. 2.

43 W. Mariner. Rationing Health Care and the Need for Credible Scarcity: Why Americans Can't Say No. *American Journal of Public Health*, 1995; 85: 1439–45.
44 J.K. Iglehart. The American Health Care System—Expenditures, op. cit., p. 70; D.M. Fox. The Politics of Trust in American Health Care. In *Ethics, Trust, and The Professions*, ed. E. Pellegrino et al. Washington, DC: Georgetown University Press, 1991.
45 For a good analysis of the variety of financial interests at stake with respect to health care spending, see, for example, Iglehart, Changing Health Insurance Trends, op. cit., pp. 956–62.
46 Chernew et al., op. cit.
47 Berk and Monheit, op. cit., pp. 9–18.
48 M. Chernew et al. Managed Care and Medical Technology: Implications for Cost Growth. *Health Affairs*, 1997; 16: 202–3; Iglehart, op cit., pp. 956–62.
49 R.H. Miller and H.S. Luft. HMO Plan Performance Update: An Analysis of the Literature, 1997–2001. *Health Affairs*, 2002; 21: 63.
50 N. Daniels. Why Saying 'No' to Patients in the U.S. is So Hard: cost-containment, Justice and Provider Autonomy. *New England Journal of Medicine*, 1986; 314: 1381–3; L. Fleck and H. Squier. Facing the Ethical Challenges of Managed Care. *Family Practice Management*, October 1995, pp. 49–55.
51 Altman and Levitt, op. cit.
52 See J. Stuart Mill. *Utilitarianism*, ed. O. Piest. Indiana: Bobbs-Merrill Educational Publishing, 1957, and P. Singer. *Writings on an Ethical Life*. New York: Harper Collins, 2000.
53 L.F. Berkman. Social Networks and Health: The Bonds that Heal. In *The Society and Population Health Reader: A State and Community Perspective*, Vol. 2, eds. A.R. Tarlov and R.F. St. Peter. New York: The Free Press, 2000, p. 260.
54 American Medical Association. *Code of Medical Ethics*, 8.13(2)b.
55 R.C. Clark. Agency Costs Versus Fiduciary Duties. In *Principles and Agents: The Structure of Business*, ed. W. Pratt and R.J. Zeckhauser. Boston: Harvard Business School Press, 1985.
56 A.A. Stone. Paradigms, Pre-emptions, and Stages: Understanding the Transformation of American Psychiatry by Managed Care. *International Journal of Law and Psychiatry*, 1995; 18: 353–87; W. Mariner. Business v. Medical Ethics: Conflicting Standards for Managed Care. *Journal of Law, Medicine and Ethics*, 1995; 23: 236–46.
57 M. Rodwin. *Medicine, Money & Morals: Physicians' Conflicts of Interest*. New York: Oxford University Press, 1993, pp. 181–4.
58 Ibid.
59 Ibid.
60 *Moore v. Regents of the University of California*, 51. 3d 120–4, 1990. But see also *D.A.B v. Brown*, 570 N.W. 2d 168 (Minn. App. 1997); *Neade v. Portes* 739 N.E. 2d 496 (ILL. 2000).
61 *Wickline v. State of California*, 727 P2d 753, 1986; P. Illingworth. A Role for Stakeholder Ethics in Meeting the Ethical Challenges Posed by Managed Care Organizations. *HEC Forum*, 1999; 11: 9–30.
62 W. Mariner. Business v. Medical Ethics: Conflicting Standards for Managed Care. *Journal of Law, Medicine and Ethics*, 1995; 23: 241; M.A. Hall et al. How Disclosing HMO Physician Incentives Affects Trust. *Health Affairs*, 2002; 21: 197–206.
63 Mariner, Business v. Medical Ethics: Conflicting Standards for Managed Care, op. cit.

64 For an alternative view of managed care's use of gag clauses, see D. Mechanic. The Managed Care Backlash: Perceptions and Rhetoric in Health Care Policy and the Potential for Health Care Reform. *Milbank Quarterly*, 2001; 79: 42.

65 Illingworth, op. cit., p. 307; J.A. Martin and L.K. Bjerknes. The Legal and Ethical Implications of Gag Clauses in Physician Contracts. *American Journal of Law and Medicine*, 1996; 22: 455–7.

66 *Dodge v. Ford Motor Co.*, Supreme Court of Michigan, 204 Mich. 459, 170 N.W. 668, 1919; Revised Model Business Code 858.30 (a), 1992; Revised Model Business Code 4.01(c); Illingworth, op. cit., p. 307.

67 Clark, op. cit., p. 73.

68 A.L. Corbin. *Corbin on Contracts*. St. Paul: West Publishing Company, 1952, p. 5.

69 *Black's Law Dictionary*, 6th ed., St. Paul: West Publishing Co., 1990, p. 322.

70 Mariner, Business vs. Medical Ethics: Conflicting Standards for Managed Care, op cit.

71 For a version of this argument grounded in ethics analysis, see E.H. Morreim. *Balancing Act: The New Medical Ethics of Medicine's New Economics*. Washington, DC: Georgetown University Press, 1995.

72 J. Sabin. The Second Phase of Priority Setting: Fairness as a Problem of Love and the Heart: A Clinician's Perspective on Priority Setting. *British Medical Journal*, 1998; 317: 1002–4.

73 Ibid.

74 N. Jecker. Dividing Loyalties: Caring for Individuals and Populations. *Yale Journal of Health Policy, Law, and Ethics*, Spring 2001; 177.

75 *Rush Prudential HMO, Inc. v. Moran*, 122 S.Ct. 2151, 2002.

76 E.H. Morreim. Moral Justice and Legal Justice in Managed Care: The Ascent of Contributive Justice. *Journal of Law, Medicine & Ethics*, 1995; 23: 247–65.

77 P.M. Nudelman and L.M. Andrews. The 'Value-Added' of Not-For-Profit Health Plans [Sounding Board]. *New England Journal of Medicine*, 1996; 334: 1057–9.

78 R. Kuttner. Must Good HMOs Go Bad? First of Two Parts: The Commercialization of Prepaid Group Health Care. *New England Journal of Medicine*, 1998; 338: 1558–63.

79 Kaiser Family Foundation, op. cit., p. 57.

80 Nudelman and Andrews, op. cit.

81 See Illingworth, op. cit., pp. 306–22.

82 P. Starr. *The Social Transformation of American Medicine*. New York: Basic Books Inc., 1982, 322.

83 Mariner, Rationing Health Care and the Need for Credible Scarcity: Why Americans Can't Say No, op. cit., pp. 1439–45.

84 Ibid.

85 Ibid.

86 N. Levinsky makes a similar point in his article, The Doctor's Master. *New England Journal of Medicine*, 1984; 311: 1757.

87 M.K. Wynia, MD, MPH, private conversation, 28 December 2002; M.K. Wynia et al. Physician Manipulation of Reimbursement Rules for Patients: Between a Rock and a Hard Place. *Journal of the American Medical Association*, 2000; 238: 1861.

88 N. Jecker. Integrating Medical Ethics with Normative Theory: Patient Advocacy and Social Responsibility. *Theoretical Medicine*, 1990; 125.

89 Ibid.

90 *Wickline v. State of California*, 192 Cal App 3d 1630, 1986.

91 H. Nelson. Non-Profit and For-Profit HMOs: Converging Practices but Different Goals? *Report of the Milbank Memorial Fund*, 1997, p. 18.

92 Jecker, op. cit.
93 Ibid.
94 R.C. Clark. Agency Costs Versus Fiduciary Duties. In *Principles and Agents: The Structure of Business*, ed. W. Pratt and R.J. Zeckhauser, Boston: Harvard Business School Press, 1985; K. Arrow. Uncertainty and the Welfare Economics of Medical Care. *American Economic Review,* 1963; III: 851–83.
95 Clark, op. cit.
96 S.J. Ellis. Rationing: Fidelity and Stewardship are Incompatible When Attempted by Same Individual. *British Medical Journal,* 1999; 318: 941.

2 Bluffing, puffing, and spinning

Health plans have been slow to disclose to patients the financial incentives they use with physicians.[1] Studies have shown that physicians deceive third-party payers to secure benefits for their patients and that patients ask their physicians to lie to their health plans.[2] In view of this, it is worth asking whether patients may eventually deceive their physicians in order to secure benefits. Could medical care be delivered in such a context? If, as some have argued, deception is commonplace in business,[3] can the truth-telling paradigm of the marketplace be imported into medicine without sacrificing too much of what is valuable in medicine? Many people believe that business organizations endorse a model of truth telling different from the one used in other contexts, and perhaps different from the one that exists in medicine.[4] As we saw in the last chapter, shareholder primacy may commit organizations to a zealous pursuit of profit maximization and to the values that ensure such profits. This is not to say that all business is 'bad' or to deny the plausibility of the popular maxim, 'doing well by doing good.'

Indeed, organizations such as the Leapfrog Group, a coalition of major U.S. companies devoted to the reduction of medical errors, are using their influence in the 'medical marketplace' to reward hospitals with their 'business.' Thus, the Leapfrog Group 'does well,' perhaps by reducing their own spending on health care and, in turn, 'doing good,' improving the safety of patients.[5] As Milstead points out, however, implementing Leapfrog Group strategies, such as computerized physician order systems, can be expensive and may involve trade-offs to, for example, hiring additional nurses.[6] But even if we grant that the characterization of business as solely motivated by profit is somewhat of a caricature, we must also acknowledge that the ethic of 'buyer beware' has a place in business that it has traditionally not had in medicine. According to some scholars, bluffing and puffing are commonplace in business and are thought to be morally sound.[7] Others believe that although deception is prevalent in business organizations, a high tolerance for deception is a fact of modern life.[8]

The question of whether health plans and the physicians who are contractually associated with them have a duty to tell the truth, has been raised directly by those concerned with whether physicians must inform patients about rationing decisions and, indirectly, by those who question the legal and ethical legitimacy of gag clauses.[9] Answers to these questions are important, not only for what they tell us about the duties of health plans and physicians, but also to tell us whether patients will themselves turn to deception in order to access care. If veracity is not strictly adhered to by health plans and the physicians who contract with them, then it is reasonable to speculate that patients, as increasingly savvy *consumers* of health care, may also resort to deception to access benefits.

The AMA states that patients have a duty to be truthful. Other than this, little attention has yet to be paid to the question of whether patients have a duty to tell the truth.[10] Would it even be desirable to encourage them to do so where the context is one in which health plans and providers routinely 'stretch' the truth?[11] Although regulations can be imposed on health plans and providers, for example to prohibit the use of gag orders and to force disclosure of financial incentives, these measures will have limited success if the underlying ethic in the health-care system is one in which bluffing, puffing, and spinning prevail. Ultimately, what is at risk is trust, the heart of the doctor–patient relationship, and the key ingredient in social capital.

Truth serves different purposes in business and medicine. It can arguably be sacrificed in the former, but not in the latter. For the purpose of evaluating truth-telling practices in managed care, I use the warranty theory of truth and argue that health plans and physicians have warranted truth. Therefore, when they deceive subscribers/patients, they do so wrongly. But this is not the only moral problem posed by the practice of manipulating the truth in a medical context. In the presence of wide-spread deception, one can speculate that patients will also lie, exacerbating problems of trust and potentially putting their own health at risk.

Bluffing and the warranty theory of truth

Deception has a variety of faces, which we view differently depending on factors such as the intent of the speaker, context, and subject matter. Because 'bluffing,' 'puffing' and 'spinning' are terms that we use on a daily basis, they have ordinary language meaning. They are also terms of art. 'Puffing' is a quasi-legal term, referring to the practice by sellers of embellishing the quality of their products.[12] When a salesperson proclaims, 'This is the best four-wheel drive on the market,' he is not making a statement of fact. He is 'puffing.' 'Bluffing' as I use it here is a term found in the field of business ethics where it is used loosely to refer to deception that occurs in a context in which the parties have consented to have the usual guarantee of truth lifted. For example, in real estate negotiations, the seller may stipulate an unreasonably high asking price knowing full well that, in this way, he will eventually get the price he wants and expects, though he was unwilling to reveal it to the buyer prior to negotiations. By withholding information, he is able to maintain the illusion that he will not budge from his asking price. 'Spin,' a term used in public relations, refers to putting a positive light on something which is potentially damaging to an organization.[13] But spin occurs in everyday contexts as well. When an investment goes sour, stockbrokers, accountants, and other 'spin doctors' are quick to highlight the tax advantages. In what follows, I will use a concept of bluffing that has appeared in the business-ethics literature. Also, in a somewhat counter-intuitive way, I will use the term 'deception' as a morally neutral term to refer to the different ways people refrain from telling the truth.

Deception is more widespread than many of us would like to acknowledge. Thus it was not surprising when President Clinton acknowledged that while under oath he made misleading, though perhaps legally accurate, statements about his relationship with Ms Lewinsky. Although many people were simply angry or disappointed with the President, others also acknowledged that sex is a subject about which people lie.[14] And still others believed that although people regularly lie about sex, they ought not to do so while under oath—that is, after they have warranted to tell the truth. Business, like politics, is a context in which arguably the rules about truth telling are relaxed and the primary oath is that of *caveat emptor*.[15] The recent Wall Street scandals, Enron and WorldCom, only confirm the rather tenuous place that truth telling has in business. Context is important for how we value instances of deception. Although not unheard of, someone who lies in the confessional still inspires puzzlement. And there may be a similar response of surprise when someone tells the truth while in the midst of negotiation with a used-car salesman.

Not atypical is Albert Carr, who supports the view that bluffing in business is ethical. He begins his defense of bluffing with a quotation from Henry Taylor, 'falsehood ceases to be falsehood when it is understood on all sides that the truth is not expected to be spoken.'[16] Carr believes that this is an accurate description of bluffing in poker, diplomacy, and business.[17] He gives the following account of his view of business bluffing:[18]

> Most executives . . . are almost compelled, in the interests of their companies or themselves, to practice some form of deception when negotiating with customers, dealers, labor unions, government officials, or even other departments of their companies. By conscious misstatements, concealment of pertinent facts, or exaggeration — in short, by bluffing — they seek to persuade others to agree with them. I think it is fair to say that if the individual executive refuses to bluff from time to time — if he feels obligated to tell the truth, the whole truth and nothing but the truth — he is ignoring opportunities permitted under the rules and is at a heavy disadvantage in his business dealings.

So bluffing is a fact of business life and business people would be at a disadvantage were they unable to bluff.[19] It is ethical, according to Carr, because no one expects otherwise. 'The game calls for distrust of the other fellow. It ignores the claim of friendship. Cunning deceptions and concealment of one's strength and intentions, not kindness and openheartedness, are vital in poker.' [20] Just as people do not judge the game of poker badly when it uses its own special brand of ethics, so they should not judge business badly for its unique brand of ethics. Thus, for Carr, bluffing in business is morally neutral.

Thomas Carson, another business ethicist, compares business bluffing to negotiations where it is to the advantage of negotiators not to reveal their minimum bargaining position.[21] He suggests a new definition of 'lying' which I call the 'warranty theory of truth.' It goes as follows: 'A lie is a false statement which the "speaker" does not believe to be true made in a context in which the speaker warrants the truth of what he says.'[22] Carson summarizes his view in the following way. 'To lie. . . is to invite trust and encourage others to believe what one says by warranting the truth of what one says and at the same time to betray that trust by making false statements which one does not believe to be true. . .'.[23] And according to Paul Ekman, 'It is not just the liar that must be considered in defining a lie, but the liar's target as well. In a lie the target has not asked to be misled, nor has the liar given any prior notification of an intention to do so.'[24]

At the heart of this view is the idea that if truth is not warranted, then it is not expected. If people are on notice that a particular context is one in which the commitment to truth telling has been relaxed, yet they nonetheless participate, then they consent. In Ekman's words they authorize the deception. This authorization transforms lying into mere bluffing and, in this way, takes the moral sting out of it. Thus consent is the relevant moral notion here. One of the implications of promising to tell the truth is that one thereby encourages others to do likewise, to tell the speaker the truth. Thus truth tellers invite others to trust them, and to tell them the truth. In view of this, people who promise to tell the truth and then renege on their promise by lying will nonetheless enjoy the truth telling their promise has encouraged. They are free riders of a sort. But just as promising to tell the truth generates truth telling, so habitual failure to tell the truth achieves the opposite. Sometimes the promise or warranty is not explicit but implicit in the context. Thus, if one party in an intimate relationship generally tells the truth, it is a betrayal of trust for the other party to lie.

Deception within health plans

If bluffing, puffing, and spinning have a role in corporate life, they may also have a presence in the business of health insurance.[25] In the corporate world, annual and quarterly reports that are required to meet security regulations are carefully designed to underplay corporate weaknesses and to highlight corporate strengths while at the same time meeting Securities and Exchange Commission disclosure requirements.[26] Advertisements make frequent use of puffing. Gag clauses certainly had the consequence of obfuscating the truth[27] and although state mandates have prohibited the use of gag clauses, there are indirect ways of manipulating information. By using cost containment mechanisms that impose a burden on truth telling and full disclosure, health plans may discourage full transparency. Practices such as economic credentialing, combined with deselection of health providers and capitation, may increase the likelihood that physicians will feel compelled to practice in a self-censored manner, both by withholding information and by avoiding high-cost medical treatment alternatives for uninformed patients.[28]

Some cost containment mechanisms indirectly interfere with their subscribers' ability to secure information. Using primary care physicians as gatekeepers can indirectly silence patients, who, aware that their physicians are uncomfortable with certain matters (sexual practices, domestic violence, family problems, drug abuse), will choose silence and forfeit their treatment.[29] In an unmanaged system, they would simply go to another physician to discuss the problem. In a managed system, however, patients may not want to antagonize their physicians, knowing that their access to care depends on the primary care physician. According to Mechanic and Schlesinger, the gatekeeper mechanism can discourage patients from communicating openly with their physicians and instead encourage them to self-censor in order to secure and maintain the goodwill of their physicians. At the same time, it will indirectly discourage them from securing the information and treatment they need for recovery.[30]

Health plans can also manipulate information with respect to the grounds they use when refusing treatment to patients. Typically, treatment is denied on the grounds that it is (1) not covered, (2) medically unnecessary, or (3) experimental. Listing specific exclusions may lend itself to comparison with other health-care organizations and this, in turn, to informed shopping, if not by subscribers, then by payers. For example, reasonable people, especially in the early days of managed care, would not have assumed that 'medically necessary' care was a term of exclusion.[31] Terms such as 'medically necessary' and 'experimental' are vague and open to interpretation and misinterpretation.[32] Vague terms fail to give notice and place a great deal of discretion in the hands of the decision-makers. From the perspective of patient welfare such discretion may be especially problematic when insurers themselves have the sole right to review appeals. Health plans can capitalize on the ambiguity of vague language to put a positive spin on the practise of denying benefits.

Puffing can be used in the advertisements of health plans. Like most corporations, health plans try to persuade consumers to purchase their services through promotional materials. To this end, they represent themselves as patient-centered, home to excellent and caring physicians, and as providers of the right care at the right time. Some important common law is developing in which the action lies in misrepresentation and breach of warranty by the health plan. In these cases managed plans have misrepresented either the quality of their service, or their primary goals in delivering services (e.g., profit v. care) in their advertisements.[33] Although the courts distinguish between mere puffing, which is permissible, and misrepresentation, which is impermissible, both are probably forms of deception.[34] But the question is of course whether they are morally permissible forms of deception? I shall argue that they are not for reasons having to do with the nature of the context. Before turning to this argument, however, I want to look at the argument that Alan Brett gives against manipulative advertising by HMOs.

Brett argues that HMOs, in particular, make liberal use of persuasive advertising. Despite the fact that persuasive advertising is standard for other products and services, he believes that it has no place in the medical context. According to Brett and others, the primary purpose of persuasive advertising is not to provide information, but to cultivate interest in a product.[35] Brett has identified four types of persuasive advertising engaged in by HMOs. First, he points out that HMO ads contradict the very purposes that guide them. One advertisement that he discusses implies that patients will have the right to see a specialist whenever they wish to, 'if you ever need the attention of one of our specialists, your private physician will refer you.'[36] Yet, the very point of a gatekeeper system is to carefully control access to costly specialists. Brett has also identified the use of manipulative language to inflate benefits, the use of exaggerated and unsubstantiated statements, and the use of irrelevant images such as sex to sell an HMO.[37]

Although these strategies are common in marketing, the conditions that may justify persuasive advertising in most cases do not, Brett argues, apply to the cases of HMOs. He explains,[38]

> Advertising by HMOs does not expand the options of most potential enrollees, and it may promote the useless movement of patients among health plans. . .whether or not such advertising influences choices, it may have secondary consequences that are undesirable, including the creation of unfair expectations among patients, the excessively commercialized portrayal of medical care, and the addition of yet another administrative expense to the health care economy.

There is little doubt that health plans, including managed ones, use manipulative advertising and in this way engage in bluffing their subscribers. Like other business organizations, MCOs employ deceptive mechanisms such as puffing and spinning on a regular basis. Brett has argued against such manipulation in the medical context. Later in this chapter, I shall do the same, but for somewhat different reasons.

Physician deception

Physicians who contract with health plans must, on the one hand, meet their fiduciary and professional duties to patients and, on the other hand, meet their contractual duties to the plan. Specifically, they have duties to provide materially beneficial care, yet may also have a contractual duty to follow cost-saving, managed-care practice guidelines. One way for them to try to deal with this conflict in duties is to deceive either patients or health plans. Haavi Morreim has discussed the possibility of physicians gaming the system at some length.[39] Gaming occurs when physicians attempt to sidestep the reimbursement rules in order to secure unintended benefits for their patients.[40] Thus gaming is an indirect way to access resources.

Physicians who game health plans may exaggerate the seriousness of a patient's condition to rationalize the ordering of tests and gain a clinically indicated, but otherwise deemed 'medically unnecessary,' hospital admission by a health plan. Physicians can also feign diagnostic uncertainty. They can specify that tests are being ordered to rule out an illness instead of as part of a routine screening in a plan that pays for the former but not the latter. In this way, they put the most favorable-to-the-patient spin on the test. From the perspective of the marketplace, this kind of exaggeration may qualify as mere puffing of the patient's condition.

There is good evidence that physicians are willing to use deception. In a recent survey undertaken by Victor G. Freeman, 70 percent of physicians surveyed by Georgetown University Medical Center indicated that they would condone lying to an insurer. According to the results of the survey the sanctioning of dishonesty was proportionately greater in areas with higher rates of managed care.[41] Research undertaken by Novack et al. also showed that physicians are willing to lie to a third-party payer to benefit patients, especially when confronted with conflicting moral values and threats to patient confidentiality.[42] In a subsequent study, Freeman et al. found that many physicians were willing to deceive third-party payers, especially when confronted with clinically severe vignettes (57.7 percent coronary bypass surgery v. 2.5 percent cosmetic rhinoplasty) and predominantly managed-care markets (40 percent of population enrolled in HMOs).[43] But the strongest evidence of physician deception comes from Matthew Wynia's study showing that roughly 40 percent of physicians manipulate reimbursement rules in order to secure benefits for their patients.[44]

Traditionally, physicians were thought to engage in paternalistic deception with patients; they kept information from patients about the seriousness of their illness for the sake of the patient,[45] and could justify doing so on the basis of the therapeutic privilege.[46] In other words, physicians have deceived patients for paternalistic reasons. Physicians have also been less than forthright with patients following their medical errors and near misses. Here the withholding of information is likely motivated by self-interest more than paternalism.[47] It is also possible for physicians to deceive patients through willful blindness about their specific plan benefits, resulting in refusal to refer them to costly specialists and limiting patient choice of providers even beyond that already limited by their health plan. Moreover, physicians can obscure from patients the financial incentives under which they are working. That is, they can ration health care implicitly and silently.[48] Implicit rationing occurs when patients are denied beneficial care for reasons having to do with the rationing of care without their knowledge. Although implicit rationing may occur because neither physician nor health plan informs the patient about rationing practices, it may also occur because though the disclosure may exist, it may be inadequate.

In one study, 101 physicians engaged in role-play responses to patient queries about how methods of compensation affected their clinical decisions.[49] The investigators found that 36 percent of physicians did not give patients enough information to allow patients to make an independent determination of how they were paid. The following are examples of the answers the physicians gave: 'My job is to be your doctor. I would not let economics change your care at all,' and 'When I first took on managed-care patients, I made a promise to myself that I would never allow it to dictate to me how I would manage patients.'[50] Even if, for the sake of argument, we were to grant that such answers are truthful, their primary purpose seems to be to reassure patients, rather than to provide them with accurate information.[51]

Deception through silence: debating disclosure

The debate over whether patients should be informed about financial incentives is puzzling, not only because of the widely recognized importance of patient self-determination, but also because truth and transparency in medicine are more widely valued today than in the past, in large part because of their importance for patient safety.[52] Even when the importance of disclosing information to patients is acknowledged, health policy scholars, who recognize the threat that explicit information about financial incentives poses for patient trust, are reluctant to impose this obligation on physicians.[53] Mandatory disclosure laws may take the matter out of the category of optional conduct.[54] In many respects, however, concerns about the disclosure of financial incentives are relics of the ethic inherent in gag clauses. At the heart of both of these policies, gag clauses and the reluctance to provide full disclosure about financial incentives and rationing practices, is a concern about how much information to give to patients about their health plans, how to deliver it, and by whom.

Mechanic and Schlesinger argue that in order to preserve trust between physician and patient, disclosure of financial incentives should be made by health plans and not physicians.[55] They state that 'Patients' trust depends on their perceptions that physicians are free to act in their best interests.'[56] If physicians are not, however, free to act in the best interest of patients, then preserving this appearance by having the information about conflicting financial incentives delivered by health plans or not at all is a form of deception. Moreover, having someone other than patients' physicians inform patients about incentives leaves patients free to believe that their own physicians will advocate for them.[57]

Elsewhere, Mechanic supports implicit rationing in which physicians assume responsibility for rationing decisions on behalf of health plans.[58] He believes that physicians are better positioned to make rationing decisions than health plan administrators, and that implicit rationing is preferable because it lowers conflict and facilitates 'stable social relations.'[59] Moreover, he recognizes that implicit rationing is often insulated from public view and that, '[d]espite the assumption that enrollees will learn about rationing processes quickly, the full implications of rationing are not likely to be salient until serious illness strikes and expensive diagnostic approaches, referrals, inpatient admissions and rehabilitative technologies are at issue.'[60]

In Hall et al.'s study on disclosure, an independent market research firm contacted plan members (1,918 subjects), initially through a letter from the plan's medical director, then through a follow-up telephone call from a market research firm.[61] The disclosure involved informing members of how their gatekeeping, primary care physicians were compensated. It also made a point of underscoring 'more of the positive features than the negative features' of the incentives.[62] Hall and Dugan found that 'with respect to knowledge of the incentives . . . the majority of subjects were still not able to correctly recall the answers to more than half of the questions.'[63] Nonetheless, the study found that disclosing the incentives under these conditions did not decrease trust in managed care physicians and health plans. Indeed, the researchers found that there was some evidence (1.4 percent) that trust increased among members of capitated plans.

Hall and Dugan et al. recognize that, although knowledge of the incentives was increased, it was still low. Given the very limited knowledge that subjects had of the incentives that the panel disclosed, it is difficult to draw any substantive conclusions about these disclosures for trust between doctor and patient. The point of disclosure, if it is to be anything but pro forma, is to ensure an understanding and appreciation of the incentives and their consequences so that members may be self-determining. Complexity of the information to be disclosed is only one of the obstacles to securing such understanding and appreciation. The apparent failure of subjects to understand the information conveyed, despite concerted effort, leads Hall et al. to speculate that, rather than attempt to convey full knowledge, it might suffice to 'provide members with the opportunity to learn about incentives if they so choose.'[64]

Surely this approach is inconsistent with the goals of informed consent. Why should lack of understanding lead to the conclusion that disclosure should be optional? First, if people do not understand the given explanations, then they may not understand that such information could be important for them. Second, it may be that plan members will not understand the implications until, as Mechanic suggests, they are seriously ill. Third, it would be interesting to know if the subjects had a choice among plans. Information about incentives may seem meaningless unless subjects can choose among plans. It may appear to them that they have no good reason to care, or that 'ignorance is bliss.' Finally, though this is purely speculative, it may be that in order for patients to arrive at a deep understanding of the financial incentives in their plans, they need to talk to their physicians. If the goal of disclosure is understanding and appreciation of both the information and its consequences, then physicians may be better equipped to effectively disclose the information.[65] Mark Hall has identified 'bundled consent' as a possible account of the consent process at work with managed plans. According to this account, subscriber consent to a managed-care plan implies consenting to all of its various details for rationing.[66] In effect, Hall believes that bundled consent at the onset of the subscriber–health-plan relationship alleviates the need to disclose *all* rationing decisions. But it is unclear that given the potentially low level of understanding, such consent could facilitate patient self-determination and autonomy.

It is important for patients to understand that the financial incentives adopted by their health plans will be implemented by their own physicians. Of course, as Mechanic points out, such disclosures by physicians may result in diminishing trust between patient and physicians at a time when such trust is especially valuable.[67] The main concern is that having health plans inform patients of financial incentives may result in manipulating information by controlling the messenger. By separating the person responsible for disclosing the information about financial incentives from physicians, we may be creating too much of an opportunity for patients to engage in a little wishful thinking. Although patients may cognitively understand the information about economic incentives (though according to Hall this is difficult), they may not appreciate the consequences of the information for their own case. That is, patients may not understand that the financial incentives mean that *their* physicians may not advocate for them as they assumed they would. There is some evidence that patients trust their physicians more than their plans.

In a recent Kaiser Harvard poll of Americans, it was found that although 52 percent polled believe that their primary care physicians will do the right thing for their care just about always, only 41 per cent believe this about their current health insurance plan.[68] Given this trust, the long fiduciary history of physicians, and the tendency of physicians to game the system and to 'lie' on behalf of their patients to third-party payers, patients may find it difficult to believe that their physicians will ration their care.[69] Unless physicians inform patients that they are personally committed to the financial incentives of the health plan and that such incentives will affect their treatment decisions and the care that patients will receive, patients may not understand this until they are seriously ill.[70] Finally, and perhaps most importantly, there is some evidence that patients want to know about the financial incentives used by their health plan. In a telephone survey of 1,050 eligible subjects, among respondents asked about cost-control bonuses, 91 percent favored disclosure of their physicians' bonuses. Furthermore, 82 percent agreed that 'I should be told whether my doctor receives a bonus without having to ask.' Many respondents also indicated concerns about asking their physicians about bonuses.[71]

It is difficult not to view the failure of health plans to voluntarily disclose financial incentives in the most effective way possible as a form of manipulation of information.[72] Moreover, if health plans were genuinely committed to transparency about incentives, they would no doubt find effective financial incentives to ensure adequate disclosure. Information about financial incentives is important for patients. Clearly, such information can help them to be better informed and more autonomous. Patients who understand the financial incentives of their plan will be better positioned to take advantage of the legal rights that they have—'the right to change PCP, to examine utilization review criteria, and to appeal coverage denials to an entity independent of the health plan.'[73] Moreover, health plans may provide better quality care in the shadow of the duty to disclose.[74] And patients may engage in more careful monitoring of their care knowing that factors other than their best interest figured into a treatment decision. Thus, even if subscribers do not have a choice among plans, information about financial incentives is important. Arguably, since the financial incentives present in a plan will affect the care that patients receive, patients require that information as much as other information they need for informed consent. Health plans that omit it, deceive patients about it, or convey the information in a way that will make it difficult for patients to fully appreciate the personal ramifications of the specifics are spinning information.

I have discussed extensively the issue of disclosing financial incentives because it is important to recognize that although 'gag' clauses are now subject to wide regulation, transparency has not become the norm. The current debate about disclosure and the reluctance of health plans to implement effective disclosure rules or to voluntarily disclose in the absence of mandates reflects the ongoing nature of the problem.[75]

Warranting the truth

Business ethicist Thomas Carson distinguishes truth from lying on the basis of what people warrant or promise. According to the warranty theory of truth, people do not lie unless they make a false statement, which they know to be false, in a context in which they have warranted to tell the truth.[76] To determine whether the 'deception' of physicians and health plans qualifies as mere bluffing or as lying, we need to ask if physicians and health plans have warranted the truth. If they have warranted the truth, yet fail to tell the truth, then their deception must count as lying.

As fiduciaries, physicians have duties of trust with respect to patients. Among their fiduciary duties are the duties to obtain informed consent and maintain patient confidentiality. Although they don't say, 'I do hereby warrant truth,' an implicit warranty can be inferred on the basis of contextual signals. Moreover, there is important case law suggesting that physicians may have duties of advocacy for their patients when cost containment mechanisms interfere with the best interest of the patient.[77] In view of these fiduciary duties, and the implicit warranty of truth telling that can be inferred from them, physicians who deceive patients, perhaps about rationing decisions, would qualify as having lied even on the warranty theory's relaxed notion of what it is to lie. An argument can also be made that health plans have warranted the truth to subscribers.[78]

Health plans that secure their subscribers through employers/payers appear to have warranted truth through the Employment Retirement Security Income Act (ERISA) and, more generally, they warrant truth through their close association with physicians who are themselves fiduciaries.[79] As I mentioned in the Introduction, ERISA is a federal act that governs employee benefits, including health-care benefits. As organizations that provide health care in addition to insurance, from the perspective of patients, health plans may have assumed some of the same fiduciary duties as physicians. Moreover, although the question of who and what has fiduciary obligations is complex, some plans will qualify as fiduciaries under ERISA.[80] ERISA imposes a number of duties on fiduciaries, including a duty to refrain from making materially false or misleading statements to plan participants.[81] In one case, an MCO was held to have violated its ERISA fiduciary duties because it had made certain misleading statements about physician incentives.[82] Whether or not a health plan will be found to be an ERISA fiduciary depends in part on the extent of discretionary power and control it exercises.[83] ERISA fiduciaries must discharge their duties 'solely in the interest of the participants and beneficiaries.'[84]

Health plans use promotional materials that promise subscribers wonderful health care with a trusting, caring physician. In these materials, they highlight their association with physicians, who have traditionally been trusted by patients,[85] and thus piggyback on that trust. Needless to say these advertisements do not mention the MCO's goal of profit maximization. Subscribers who receive their health care through their employment may also transfer to their health plan the trust they have for their employer. Moreover, employers who provide their employees with health plans through self-insured mechanisms may also incur certain ERISA-based fiduciary obligations to their employees.

Health plans may also warrant the truth through their affiliation with various professional associations. For example, the American Association of Health Plans (AAHP) represents over 1,000 plans, serving 170 million Americans. The organization serves a variety of managed plans including

HMOs and PPOs. According to their Philosophy of Care, they 'are committed to high standards of quality and professional ethics, and to the principle that patients come first.' With respect to information the AAHP says, 'We believe that consumers have a right to information about health plans and how they work.'[86] In a section devoted specifically to patient information, the Code of Conduct states that 'health plans have pledged to ensure that each patient has access to all information . . . required to promote the right care.'[87] These various 'commitments' and 'pledges' would seem to constitute a warrant to tell the truth, at least for those 1,000 plans affiliated with the AAHP.

A strong case can be made that both health plans and physicians have warranted the truth. Thus, according to the warranty theory of truth, when they use deception they do so unethically; they lie. Lying is wrong here because it violates the warranty theory of truth, and it creates a context in which it is difficult for the truth to be told. If health plans and physicians lie to each other and to patients, they create a climate in which patients may believe that they have little choice but to lie as well. If patient deception is fostered in this way, it only compounds the wrong inherent in violating the warranty theory of truth.

Patient deception: damned if they do, damned if they don't

At this time, we do not have any studies documenting an increase in patient deception. This is not to say that such deception does not exist. There is certainly anecdotal evidence of patient deception. Nonetheless, any comments that I make about patient deception must necessarily be speculative. I shall approach this question by considering whether (1) patients could deceive their physicians, and (2) it makes sense from their perspective to do so. With respect to (1) there is good evidence that today some patients are more active and better informed about their medical care than they were in the past.[88] Increasingly, patients are referred to as 'consumers.' This language may signal a shift both in how patients are viewed and what expectations we have of them. Their enhanced knowledge base may be a result of increased access to information technology. But it also comes at a time, as Kassirer points out, when patients are dissatisfied with the doctor–patient relationship and have become accustomed to impersonal interactions with their physicians.[89] Certainly, if patients choose to deceive their physicians there are opportunities to do so; they could malinger, pretend to have symptoms that they do not have, or trump up symptoms with an eye to securing referrals to specialists or expensive tests and medications. That is, they could game the system as physicians have.[90]

In order for patients to deceive effectively, they would need to know enough about symptoms, diagnosis, and treatments to make their deception plausible. Today patients have access to an enormous and unprecedented amount of medical information on the Internet. The results of a recent survey conducted by the Pew Internet and American Life Project suggested that 55 percent of U.S. internet users have sought health information on the Internet, about 52 million Americans.[91] In another 2000 survey, researchers found that 91 percent of 'health seekers' were looking for information about a physical illness and 26 percent about a mental illness.[92] There was a 200 percent increase in consumer use of Medline after 1997, when the National Library of Medicine made it available to the public. The public constituted 30 percent of total Medline use—a jump from 10 percent.[93]

Patient activism has also been facilitated by recent changes to the rules governing the advertising of drugs directly to patients. In August 1997, the Food and Drug Administration liberalized its guidelines for direct-to-consumer advertising for drugs to permit television advertising. This makes it easier for pharmaceutical companies to target patients directly and, in turn, supplements patients' information about drugs. Direct-to-consumer advertising is credited with increasing pharmaceutical sales and may drive patients to the doctor's office with a desire for expensive drugs and often unrealistic expectations.[94] Although many physicians are skeptical about 'Internet medicine' and the information patients obtain from the Internet, many also recognize that patients are better informed about some illnesses than are some treating physicians.[95] At most, this evidence of patient as consumer establishes that many patients have the wherewithal to deceive their physicians. That is, they have the informational savvy to deceive them should they decide to.

Psychiatrists are familiar with the many different ways that patients deceive their physicians. Munchausen syndrome, malingering and imposters are illustrative of the kinds of patient deception they encounter in their practice.[96] In a report of the *Journal of the American Medical Association* it was noted that online support groups have proven to be a haven for people who pretend to have an illness in order to secure sympathy and nurturing.[97] Moreover, the report underscores that online information 'makes it easy for people faking an illness to get details about their supposed condition.'[98] Although it isn't clear from the report whether or not the Internet has fostered more patient deception, it does explicitly say that it is easier for patients to lie now than in the past. Patients may not now be lying to their physicians, but in the face of continuous erosion of the relationship between doctor and patient, they may do so in the future.[99] The crux of the problem is that as the fiduciary component of the doctor–patient relationship is eroded, we can anticipate that the behavior of patients may change accordingly.

Patients may decide to live up to the name 'consumer,' and adopt a *caveat emptor* approach to the doctor–patient relationship. We do know from Wynia et al.'s study that patients frequently ask their physicians to lie to third-party payers for them.[100] Another survey conducted in 1998–99 found that most consumers (70 percent of those surveyed) believe that doctors put medical needs first.[101] Patients who choose not to deceive their physicians may believe that they do not need to lie because physicians are continuing to advocate for them. But what if that changes and patients no longer believe that their physicians will act in their interest? If the trend to view patients as consumers continues to gain ground, and if patients begin to view themselves as consumers, they may in turn adopt the values and actions of consumers. One common justification that people give for lying to others is that they have been the victim of a lie.[102] Psychologically there is an easing of standards of truthfulness once people have been lied to such that they have fewer reservations about lying. Morally, rightly or wrongly, once people have been lied to they may invoke the principle of 'a lie for a lie.'[103] Given this principle, diminished trust between doctor and patient, one can speculate that the presence of gaming, bluffing, puffing and spinning in the medical context may serve as an invitation and rationalization for patients to lie.[104]

In a context in which some beneficial care may be denied, patients may believe that they will increase their chances of securing medical care if they deceive their physicians. Just as physicians have demonstrated a willingness to deceive third-party payers to secure health care for their patients,[105] so in the absence of trust between doctor and patient, patients may find that they are willing to deceive their physicians to secure their own care. If the bond of trust between patient and physician is eroded, then one important barrier to patient deception may have thereby been lifted. Put differently, if patients cum consumers were to view their physicians as the mere providers of a service, some of the reason for maintaining trust and, in turn, a high level of truth telling, will have dissipated.[106] Studies show that people lie on a regular basis in everyday conversations. Robert S. Feldman found that 60 percent of people lied at least one time during a ten-minute conversation and, on average, two or three times. According to Feldman, lying is part of daily living.[107] In the absence of a bond of trust, the conversations between doctors and patients may assume the character of everyday conversations and include the relatively low standard of truth telling of these conversations. Fiduciary duties may contribute to truth telling both directly, by requiring physicians to tell the truth (informed consent), and indirectly, by creating a context in which patients are invited to rise above everyday truth-telling practices and encouraged to tell the truth.

The consequences of patient deception would be substantial. It is difficult, if not impossible in some cases, for physicians to make accurate and timely diagnoses if patients deceive them about symptoms, etc. Thus patients find themselves trapped between the proverbial rock and hard place—damned if they do and damned if they don't. From their point of view, they may have nothing to gain from truth telling, but something to gain from deception (even if not in the end their health). Moreover, implicit rationing of this kind, endorsed by Mechanic, would be close to impossible if patients tried to manipulate their physicians. As Mechanic states, '[i]mplicit rationing works because patients trust that doctors are their agents and have their interests at heart.'[108]

Mechanic has discussed some of the losses to patients when there is a breakdown in trust. Trust ensures a high quality of communication between doctor and patient. This, in turn, makes it more likely that patients will discuss personal information about stigmatized conditions, cooperate with treatment, and adopt health-promoting behavior.[109] Norman Levinsky points out that when rationing decisions are not disclosed to patients they are thereby deprived of the right to contest the decision to ration care in their own case—and as a social policy.[110] Patients have too much to lose through deception. Finally, patients may be too sick to deceive their physicians effectively. Successful deception requires a good memory, while many illnesses involve memory impairment. Deception requires a level of effort that many sick patients may not be capable of. When physicians and health plans lie, they increase the likelihood that patients will lie. But when patients lie, they put their health at risk. Deception in health plans puts patients at increased risk of harm from the consequences of the deception.

Assumption of the risk

It might be argued that if patients engage in deception themselves, they would not be entitled to object to the harms that befall them. In other words, although patients may be harmed by any deception they engage in, they assume the risk associated with it. But an assumption of the risk argument of this kind requires that patients voluntarily assume the risk. Patients don't choose to be sick and they often don't have much choice about their health-care plans. Rightly or wrongly, they may believe that they stand to lose their health and even their lives, if they do not deceive their providers. Moreover, the presence of a context in which deception is widespread increases the likelihood that patients will deceive their physicians and in this way undermine their own care. Given these conditions, it would be difficult to construe either patient deception as voluntarily engaged in, or the harms associated with it, as voluntarily assumed.

Business ethicists like Carr and Carson believe that bluffing is widespread in business and recent Wall Street scandals bear this out. Like other business organizations, health plans may be making liberal use of deceptive mechanisms. Unlike other business organizations, however, they do so in a context that has a long fiduciary history, in which the main participants do not anticipate deception and cannot in any case consent to the deception. As we shall see in the next chapter, trust between doctor and patient is at risk.[111] In view of this, it is reasonable to anticipate that deception will continue, if not increase. Nonetheless, a lie is a lie and not a bluff.

The warranty theory of truth may be right when it asserts that one needs to have warranted truth in order for a falsehood to count as a lie. In this way, the theory highlights the moral significance of context. Medical care depends on patients telling the truth and what the warranty theory high-lights is that it is difficult for patients to tell the truth when other significant parties lie. It might be argued that patients have a self-interested reason to tell the truth, their health. That is, they believe that telling the truth will facilitate diagnosis, treatment, and care. But in the world of aggressively managed medical care, many patients may not believe that their physicians and health plans have their interests at heart or will be forthcoming with the resources they believe are necessary.[112] In these circumstances there may be less of an incentive for patients to tell the truth. Apparent self-interest, combined with diminished trust, may lead patients to deceive their providers.

Managed medical care may foster deception within the world of health care. It is still unclear, for example, whether some form of deception about financial incentives is necessary in order for managed care to be viable. David Mechanic believes that patients should not be informed about rationing, and especially not by their physicians, because to do so would put trust at risk and trust seems to be an essential component of medi-cine.[113] Mark Hall seems to believe that trust is not at risk from disclosure; yet the subjects of his study had low comprehension of the incentives and in any case were not informed by their doctors. But the question remains, 'What will happen to the doctor–patient relationship if there is complete transparency about the incentives used by managed care?' Widespread deception has the potential to harm patients, not only by creating a climate in which patients may themselves lie, but also by depleting the reservoir of trust that has traditionally existed between doctor and patient.

Notes

1 T.E. Miller and W.M. Sage. Disclosing Physician Financial Incentives. *Journal of the American Medical Association*, 1999; 281: 1424–30.
2 M.K. Wynia et al. Physician Manipulation of Reimbursement Rules for Patients: Between a Rock and a Hard Place. *Journal of the American Medical Association*, 2000; 238: 1858–65.
3 J. Useem. Should you lie? *Fortune Small Business*, November 1999; J. Kurlantzick, Liar, Liar. *Entrepreneur Magazine*, October 2003, pp. 68–71.
4 J. Useem, op. cit.; A.Z. Carr, Is Business Bluffing Ethical? In *Ethical Theory and Business*, 5th edn, ed. T.L. Beauchamp and N.E. Bowie. New Jersey: Prentice Hall, 1997, pp. 451–6; T. Carson. Second Thoughts About Bluffing. In Beauchamp and Bowie, op. cit., pp. 456–62.
5 J.A. Milstead. Leapfrog Group: A Prince in Disguise or Just Another Frog? *Nursing Administration Quarterly*, 2002; 26: 16–25.
6 Ibid.
7 Carr, op. cit.; Carson, op. cit.
8 Kurlantzick, op. cit.
9 See N.G. Levinsky. Truth or Consequences. *New England Journal of Medicine*, 1998; 338: 913–15; J.A. Martin and L.K. Bjerknes. The Legal and Ethical Implications of Gag Clauses in Physician Contract. *American Journal of Law and Medicine*, 1996; 22: 433–76; M.A. Hall. Informed Consent to Rationing

Decisions. *Milbank Quarterly*, 1993; 71: 645–67; D. Mechanic. The Managed Care Backlash: Perceptions and Rhetoric in Health Care Policy and the Potential for Health Care Reform. *Milbank Quarterly*, 2001; 79: 42–44.

10 American Medical Association Council on Ethical and Judicial Affairs. *Code of Medical Ethics Current Opinions and Annotations*, 10.02. Chicago: AMA Press, 2002.

11 Although M. Benjamin's work is useful on questions concerning the foundation of patients' obligations to their physicians, it speaks only briefly to the question that concerns this chapter—what patients ought to do when medical professionals and providers engage in deception. Benjamin's position is consistent with contract law, namely, that breach of obligation by one party releases the other party from having to meet their obligations. See: M. Benjamin. Lay Obligations in Professional Relations. *Journal of Medicine and Philosophy*, 1985; 10: 85–103; Wynia et al., op. cit. For an article on how MCOs manipulate the truth, see A.S. Brett. The Case Against Persuasive Advertising by Health Maintenance Organizations. *New England Journal of Medicine*, 1992; 326: 1353–6.

12 *Black's Law Dictionary*, 6th ed. St Paul: West Publishing Co., 1990, p. 1233.

13 S. Ewen. *PR! A Social History of Spin*. New York: Basic Books, 1996.

14 D. Duggan. Let's Keep Sex Behind Closed Doors. *Newsday*, 15 November 1998, Queens ed.

15 It is not my intention to overstate this point. That is, I am not claiming that everyone in business and management lies. There are obviously many honest and ethical people in the world of business.

16 Carr, op. cit., p. 451.

17 Ibid.

18 Ibid.

19 B. Horowitz. When Should Executives Lie? *Industrial Week*, 16 November 1981.

20 Carr, op. cit., p. 454.

21 Carson, op. cit.

22 Ibid., p. 459.

23 Ibid.

24 P. Ekman. *Telling Lies*. New York: W.W. Norton and Company Inc., 1992, p. 27.

25 Useem, op. cit.

26 *Backman v. Polaroid Corporation*, 910 F. 2d 10 (1st Cir. 1990).

27 Mechanic, op. cit., pp. 35–54.

28 Levinsky, op. cit., p. 914; S. Woolhandler and D.U. Himmelstein. Extreme Risk—The New Corporate Proposition for Physicians. *New England Journal of Medicine*, 1995; 334: 1706–9; D. Mechanic and M. Schlesinger. The Impact of Managed Care on Patients' Trust in Medical Care and Their Physicians. *Journal of the American Medical Association*, 1996; 275: 1696.

29 Mechanic and Schlesinger, op. cit., p. 1695.

30 Ibid.

31 W.K. Mariner. Business vs. Medical Ethics: Conflicting Standards for Managed Care. *Journal of Law, Medicine and Ethics*, 1995; 23: 241.

32 D.M. Eddy. Benefit Language. *Journal of the American Medical Association*, 1996, 275: 650; some of the vagueness in the language of, for example, medical necessity, may be clarified. The settlements between Aetna and a number of physicians focused in part on Aetna's agreement to clarify the meanings of these terms. J.B. Treaster. Aetna Agreement With Doctors Envisions Altered Managed Care. *The New York Times*, 23 May 2000. Late ed-final, section A, p. 1, col. 1.

33 See *McClellan v. Health Maintenance Org. of Pennsylvania*, 604 A2d 1053 (Pa. Sup. Ct 1992) (finding ostensible agency based on advertisements by the HMO and claiming that it carefully screened primary care physicians).

34   This point underscores the crux of the problem. Puffing is an acceptable and legally permissible part of business. Yet, in the medical context it is highly problematic in part because the medical context has a long tradition of fiduciary relationships and because the success of the doctor–patient relationship depends on truth.

35   Brett, op. cit., p. 1354; T.L. Beauchamp. Manipulative Advertising. In Beauchamp and Bowie, op. cit., pp. 472–80.

36   Brett, op. cit., p. 1354.

37   Ibid.

38   Ibid., p. 1356.

39   E.H. Morreim. *Balancing Act: The New Medical Ethics of Medicine's New Economics.* Washington, DC: Georgetown University Press, 1995, pp. 70–2.

40   Ibid., p. 70.

41   V.G. Freeman. Liar, Liar—the Pinocchio Dilemma. *Modern Physician*, August 1997, p. 6.

42   D.H. Novack et al. Physicians' Attitudes Toward Using Deception to Resolve Difficult Ethical Problems. *Journal of the American Medical Association*, 1998; 261: 2983.

43   V.G. Freeman et al. Lying for Patients: Physician Deception of Third Party Payers. *Archives of Internal Medicine*, 1999; 159: 2263–70.

44   Wynia et al., op. cit., p. 1861.

45   H. Spire. *The Power of Hope.* New Haven: Yale University Press, 1998, pp. 111–18.

46   Evidence for this can be found in the recent incident involving a physician who left his patient in the midst of complex surgery to go to the bank. After the physician was suspended, a decision was made not to inform the patient about the transfer of care until he had adequately convalesced. M. Romano. Loophole Tied to Bizarre Case. *Modern Healthcare*, 19 August 2000, p. 10.

47   A.W. Wu et al. How House Officers Cope with Their Mistakes. *Western Journal of Medicine*, 1993, 159: 5565–69; Novack et al., op. cit., pp. 2980–5; D. Hilfiken. Facing Our Mistakes. *New England Journal of Medicine*, 1984; 310: 118–22.

48   Some might argue that implicit rationing is not a form of deception. However, given the amount of discussion and analysis in the scholarly literature over whether or not physicians should inform patients about incentives, it is difficult at this point to view the omission as other than intentional manipulation of information. See, for example, D. Mechanic. Models of Rationing: Professional Judgment and the Rationing of Medical Care, 140 University of Pennsylvania Law Review, May 1992, pp. 1713–54.

49   S.D. Pearson and T. Hyams. Talking About Money: How Primary Care Physicians Respond to a Patient's Questions About Financial Incentives. *Journal of General Internal Medicine*, 2002; 17: 75–8.

50   Ibid.

51   Ibid., p. 77.

52   The Institute of Medicine. *President's Report to the Members*, 16 October 2001 Annual Meeting. Online, available at <http://www.iom.edu> (accessed 2003); F. Rosmer et al. Disclosure and the Prevention of Medical Errors. *Archives of Internal Medicine*, 2000; 160: 2089–92; L. Leape. Error in Medicine. *Journal of the American Medical Association*, 1994; 272: 1851–7; H. Talfryn Oakley Davies and M. Neil Marshall. Public Disclosure of Performance Data: Does the Public Get What the Public Wants? *The Lancet*, 1999; 353: 1639–40; S. Pinker. Quebec Moves Toward Full Disclosure of Medical Errors. *CMAJ-JAMC*, 2002; 166: 800; J. Jones. CMS Attacked over Delay in Reducing Secrecy. *British Medical Journal*, 2000; 321: 135.

53 Mechanic. Models of Rationing: Professional Judgment and the Rationing of Medical Care, op. cit.
54 T. Miller and W. Sage. Disclosing Physician Financial Incentives. *Journal of the American Medical Association*, 1999; 281: 1424–30; *Pegram v. Herdrich*, 536 U.S. 355 2000.
55 Mechanic and Schlesinger, op. cit., pp. 1696–7.
56 Ibid. As we shall see in Chapter 3, this corresponds to what Hardin and I refer to as trust based on encapsulated interest.
57 This would seem to follow from what Mechanic says in the following about the inability of patients to understand the implication of managed care. Mechanic. Models of Rationing: Professional Judgment and the Rationing of Medical Care, op. cit.; D. Mechanic and M. Schlesinger. Professionalism in Medicine: Can Patients Trust in Managed Care? *Journal of the American Medical Association*, 1996; 276: 951.
58 Mechanic. Models of Rationing: Professional Judgment and the Rationing of Medical Care, op. cit.
59 D. Mechanic. Dilemmas in Rationing Health Care Services: The Case for Implicit Rationing. *British Medical Journal*, 1995; 310: 1655–9.
60 Mechanic. Models of Rationing: Professional Judgment and the Rationing of Medical Care, op. cit.
61 The connection between disclosure and trust was studied by Hall et al., see M.A. Hall et al. How Disclosing HMO Physician Incentives Affects Trust. *Health Affairs*, 2002; 197–206.
62 Ibid.
63 Ibid.
64 Ibid.
65 Ibid.
66 M. Hall. Informed Consent to Rationing Decisions. *Milbank Quarterly*, 2003; 71: 645–68.
67 Mechanic and Schlesinger. The Impact of Managed Care on Patients' Trust in Medical Care and Their Physicians, op. cit., pp. 1693–7; Mechanic. Models of Rationing: Professional Judgment and the Rationing of Medical Care, op. cit.
68 Kaiser Family Foundation/Harvard School of Public Health. National Survey of Consumer Experiences With and Attitudes Toward Health Plans, August 2001. See also Kao's finding that regardless of payment method, patients had less trust for their health plans than their physicians, A.C. Kao et al. The Relationship Between Method of Physician Payment and Patient Trust. *Journal of the American Medical Association*, 1998; 280: 1708–14.
69 Morreim, op. cit.; Wynia et al., op. cit.
70 D. Mechanic and S. Meyer. Concepts of Trust Among Patients with Serious Illness. *Social Science and Medicine*, 2000; 51: 657–68.
71 T.H. Gallagher et al. Patients' Attitudes Toward Cost Control Bonuses for Managed Care Physicians. *Health Affairs*, 2001; 20: 189.
72 U.S. General Accounting Office. *Consumer Health Care Information: Many Quality Commission Recommendations Are Not Current Practice*. Washington, DC: General Accounting Office, 1998.
73 T.E. Miller and W.M. Sage. Disclosing Physician Financial Incentives. *Journal of the American Medical Association*, 1999; 281: 1427.
74 Ibid., pp. 1424–30.
75 State mandates do not apply to the many self-insured plans used primarily by large employers; ibid.
76 T. Carson. Second Thoughts About Bluffing. In *Ethical Theory and Business*, 5th edn, ed. T.L. Beauchamp and N.E. Bowie. New Jersey: Prentice Hall, 1997, pp. 456–62.

77 *Wickline v. State of California*, 192 Cal. App 3d 1630, 1986.
78 See Mariner, op. cit.
79 ERISA, 1974, 88 Stat. 832, 29 U.S.C. 1001–1461.
80 ERISA, 1974, § 3(21)(A), 29 U.S.C; § 1002(21)(A).
81 *Varity Corp. v. Howe*, 516 U.S. 489, 1996.
82 *Drolet v. Healthsource*, 968 F. Supp., 757, 1997. But see also *Ehlman v. Kaiser Foundation Healthplans of Texas*, 198 T. 3d 552 (5th Circ. 2000).
83 "[A] person is a fiduciary with respect to a plan to the extent: The person exercises any discretionary authority or discretionary control respecting management of such plan or exercises any authority or control respecting management disposition of its assets. (ERISA 3(21)(a) of ERISA, 29 U.S.C. § 1002(21)(a))."
84 ERISA, 1974, § 404(a)(1).
85 M. Hall. Trust, Law and Medicine. *Stanford Law Review*, 2002; 55: 463–527; U.S.A. Today/CNN/Gallup Poll, 5–8 July 2002, as described in J.M. Jones. Poll Analyses: Americans Express Little Trust in CEOs of Large Corporations or Stockbrockers. *Gallup News Service*, 17 July 2002; Mechanic and Schlesinger. The Impact of Managed Care on Patients' Trust in Medical Care and Their Physicians, op. cit.
86 American Association of Health Plans. *Philosophy of Care*. Online, available at <http://www.aahp.org> (accessed 2003).
87 American Association of Health Plans. *Code of Conduct*. Online, available at <http://www.aahp.org> (accessed 2003).
88 J. Kassirer. Patients, Physicians, and the Internet. *Health Affairs*, 2000; 19: 117.
89 Ibid., pp. 116–19.
90 Wynia et al., op. cit.; Morreim, op. cit.
91 LNT. Internet Use Affects Health Care Decision-Making, Survey Confirms: Information Seekers Don't Divulge Personal Data. *American Journal of Health-System Pharmacy*, 2001; 58: 107–8.
92 Ibid.
93 T. Leaffer and B. Gonda. The Internet: An Underutilized Tool in Patient Education. *Computers in Nursing*, 2000; 18: 47–52.
94 See W. Zachry et al. Relationship Between Direct-to-Consumer Advertising and Physician Diagnosing and Prescribing. *American Journal of Health-System Pharmacy*, 2002; 59: 42–9; D. Young. Studies Show Drug Ads Influence Prescription Decisions, Drug Costs. *American Journal of Health-System Pharmacy*, 2002; 59: 14, 16.
95 Kassirer, op. cit., pp. 116–19.
96 H.K. Gediman and J.S. Lieberman. *The Many Faces of Deceit*. New Jersey: Jason Aronson Inc., 1996, pp. 21–3.
97 J. Stephenson. Patient Pretenders Weave Tangled 'Web' of Deceit. *Journal of the American Medical Association*, 1998; 280: 1297.
98 Ibid.
99 D. Lupton et al. Caveat Emptor or Blissful Ignorance? Patients and the Consumerist Ethos. *Social Science and Medicine*, 1991; 33: 559–68.
100 Wynia et al., op. cit.
101 J. Lee Hargraves. *Data Bulletin Number 17*. Washington, DC: Center for Studying Health System Change, 2000.
102 S. Bok. Lying to Liars. In *Lying*. London: Quartet Books Limited, 1978, pp. 123–33.
103 Ibid.
104 In managed plans, patients may be denied care they believe they need. Lying may seem to them the best way to secure their care. Since Wynia's study shows that patients are prepared to ask their physicians to lie to third party payers on

their behalf, we can infer that they know that lying is an effective way to get benefits. The question is would they be willing to lie to their physician if and when they come to believe that their physicians are withholding care and will not game the system on their behalf. Wynia et al., op. cit.

105 Ibid.
106 For an interesting discussion about this in the Australian and British context, see Lupton et al., op. cit.
107 R.S. Feldman et al. Self-Presentation and Verbal Deception: Do Self-Presenters Lie More? *Journal of Basic and Applied Social Psychology*, 2002; 24: 163–70.
108 D. Mechanic. Dilemmas in Rationing Health Care Services: The Case for Implicit Rationing, op. cit.
109 D. Mechanic. Changing Medical Organization and the Erosion of Trust. *Milbank Quarterly*, 1996; 74: 177.
110 Levinsky, op. cit.
111 U.S.A. Today/CNN/Gallup Poll, 5–8 July 2002, as described in Jones, op. cit.
112 Kaiser Family Foundation/Harvard School of Public Health, op. cit.
113 Mechanic. Models of Rationing: Professional Judgment and the Rationing of Medical Care, op. cit.

3 Trust: the scarcest of medical resources

Truth and trust go hand in hand.[1] When truth is compromised, trust may be sacrificed. Given the potential for bluffing, puffing, and spinning in health care, it is not surprising that trust between doctor and patient has been adversely affected. The potential for patients to trust their health plans, doctors and the institution of medicine itself may be impaired by managed care.[2] Moreover, scholars are aware of the importance of trust for the doctor–patient relationship and, in turn, the need for health plans to monitor its loss.[3] Concern about compromised trust between doctor and patient has led some scholars to search for alternatives to the trust of the traditional doctor–patient relationship.[4] At the time of writing, some empirical studies show that trust in physicians has diminished only slightly,[5] and that the public is concerned about managed-care plans.[6] However, it would be a mistake to assume from this that trust between patient and physician is infinitely robust. Given what we know about trust between doctor and patient, it is predictable that if the doctor–patient relationship continues to be stressed, trust will continue its downward slide.

Although trust is in general a moral and social good, loss of trust could be arguably tolerated on the basis of the ethics of contract. By invoking a consent argument, according to which free and autonomous subscribers choose their own plans and the doctor–patient relationships that go with them, it could be argued that they prefer lower-priced and lower-trust doctor–patient relationships.[7] In this way, a loss of trust can be spun into a celebration of patient autonomy. Despite these attempts to find the 'silver lining,' there are good reasons not to relegate this matter to the sphere of private harm, freely chosen by supposedly 'rugged patients.'[8] The problem is that diminished trust from the doctor–patient relationship may very well entail costs that are borne not only by patients, who in a fictional world freely choose lower-trust health plans, but also by the community.[9] When we look at trust as a form of social capital, focusing on the role that it plays in social well-being, and the paucity of opportunities available for its cultivation, it can be argued that trust cultivation should not be left in the hands of organizations that are concerned primarily with a narrowly defined set of interests—shareholder welfare.

In this chapter, I provide a conceptual definition of 'trust' and show how, given this understanding, trust is unlikely to flourish in aggressively managed health plans that place excessive pressure on the doctor–patient relationship. This account of trust overlaps in substantive ways with some of the characteristics that David Mechanic has observed as important for patients who trust their physicians.[10] The virtue of the conceptual model that I use is that it can be used to predict the effect of different kinds of conduct or policy on the cultivation of trust and social capital. I also discuss some of the empirical studies and surveys of trust.

Although neither of these approaches show with certainty that managed care has undermined trust in the doctor–patient relationship, together they provide a powerful reason to be concerned about the future of medical trust. Before turning to that discussion, a caveat is in order. To say that some aggressively implemented managed-care practices put trust between doctor and patient at risk is not to say that all managed care is unconcerned with trust. Certainly the efforts of the National Committee for Quality Assurance (NCQA), including both accreditation of HMOs and the measurement and publication of quality both endorsed and used by a number of HMOs, are bound to contribute positively to patient trust. Nevertheless, these steps, though valuable, may not be sufficient to counteract the harmful effects of some practices.[11] Although some large corporations, such as Xerox and IBM, make accreditation a requirement of their health plans, most employers do not. Publication of Health Plan Employer Data and Information Set (HEDIS) data, though helpful to consumers in assessing the performance of managed health plans, is not mandatory, and those who choose not to publicize their HEDIS profile are those with lower scores.[12]

Later in this chapter, I also look at potential counter-arguments to the view that I develop. The first argument maintains that there is no reason to worry about trust between doctor and patient because, although trust is valuable, trust between doctor and patient is uniquely resilient.[13] The second counter-argument minimizes the significance of trust between doctor and patient and instead suggests that it be replaced with trustworthy institutions that follow fair procedures.

My own view is that trust between doctor and patient is indeed valuable, not only because of the benefits it confers on the patient, but because of the benefits it confers on the community. I will argue that because trust in organizations is less 'rich' than interpersonal trust, theories that advocate replacing trust between doctor and patient with trust in organizations will ultimately deplete an important source of trust for the community.

Trust

There is widespread concern that implementation of the most aggressive forms of managed care carries with it losses—to both the quality of medical care and the doctor–patient relationship.[14] At risk is the trust that has traditionally flourished between doctor and patient.[15] Trust can be defined in a number of ways.[16] Russell Hardin points out that trust involves a three-part relationship.[17] When we talk about 'trust', we say 'A trusts B to do Y.'[18] That is, we rarely have global or generalized trust for people. Instead, we trust them with respect to certain activities or expectations. In this respect, trust is context-based.

In addition to context, Hardin identifies two conceptual factors that are needed to understand 'trust.' In the first, the 'encapsulated interest' account, trust is to be understood in terms of the interest of the trustee (the person trusted) in being trustworthy. That is, the entruster (the person doing the trusting) is able to develop confidence in the trustee because he knows that it is in the interest of the trustee to act in ways that are consistent with that trust. For example, there may be a profitable, long-term business relationship between the two that ensures that it is in the interest of the trustee to be trustworthy. In this view, trust is possible because trustworthiness is the rational course for the trustee to take.[19] Second, the 'economic' or 'Bayesian' theory of trust focuses on the individual believer and how she comes to believe in the trustworthiness of others.[20] Hardin suggests the use of a street-level epistemology that looks at how people's childhoods and limited information about the world affect their ability to trust.[21] Here, individual experience determines people's capacity to trust. Depending on their experience, people have higher and lower capacities to trust. Thus the capacity to trust is learned and presumably modified throughout a person's life.[22]

Trust can also be 'thick' or 'thin.' Thick trust is found in relationships that are frequent, strong, and personal, such as those between a resident and her postman. Thin trust is extended to new acquaintances and is often based on a generalized reciprocity and mutual expectations. Thin trust is extremely valuable, especially in a diverse society, because it extends trust, and the benefits that flow from it, from small insular groups to larger diverse groups.[23]

Both the encapsulated and economic conceptions of trust are relevant to our understanding of how trust is created and maintained in the doctor–patient relationship. What patients believe about their physicians' motives will be one ingredient in determining their level of trust, but it will not be the only one. Factors having to do with individual histories, past experiences with the health-care system, physicians and others will also affect trust levels. According to David Mechanic, trust is difficult to come by and fragile.[24] Its acquisition requires repeated trust-producing events; yet, trust that has taken years to build can be dashed with one trust-destroying incident.[25] The two prongs of Hardin's account treat trust as contingent largely on the beliefs of entrusters. Thus trust is evidence-based. For example, if a patient believes that it is in the interest of her physician to be trustworthy, she will be more likely to trust.

Support for this evidence-based approach to trust can also be found in a study undertaken by Mechanic and Meyer of 90 seriously ill patients. They found that patients regularly engage in testing their physicians as they decide whether to trust them.[26] When Mechanic and Meyer interviewed patients with serious illnesses about trust, they found that the most common themes patients articulated were concerns with 'honesty, openness, responsiveness, having one's best interest at heart, and willingness to be vulnerable without fear of being harmed.'[27] They also found that although some patients take the 'trustworthy until proven otherwise' attitude, most commonly patients are involved in testing their physicians against their expectations to determine their trustworthiness.[28] A focus-group study conducted by Thom and Campbell also showed some common threads. Although the study revealed that patients identified nine dimensions of trust, patients attributed special importance to physician rapport, compassion, understanding, and honesty.[29] In a later study conducted by Thom, it was found that the physician behaviors most strongly associated with trust were (1) being comforting and caring, (2) demonstrating competence, (3) encouraging and answering questions, (4) explaining what they were doing, and (5) referring to a specialist if needed.[30] A similar theme of honesty, openness, and transparency appears in the studies of both Mechanic and Thom.

These patients' reports are consistent with Hardin's approach to trust. Patient concern with physicians who are honest and open could reflect a desire for transparency about the interests of the physician, buttressing Hardin's encapsulated interest account. Concern by patients about whether physicians will act in their best interest, or have one's best interest at heart, may be a strategy to assess what other physician interests may be operating. That is, patients may be trying to rule out physician interests that are inconsistent with trustworthy behavior. Furthermore, the fact that patients typically observe and test their physician's trustworthiness suggests that, for patients, trust is a cognitive process, based on evidence for or against their beliefs.

Of course, if Hardin's account of trust is right, patients may fail to trust even the most trustworthy of physicians because (a) patients are unable to believe that it is in the interest of the physician to be trustworthy or (b) their capacity to trust has been compromised because they have had too many trust-diminishing experiences. Thus the physician's behavior or invitation to trust is only one part of the evidentiary framework that patients use to formulate their set of beliefs about their physicians. If trust is a primarily cognitive process, then trustworthy physicians who work for untrustworthy health-care organizations or who are subject to conflicts of interest are vulnerable to being regarded as untrustworthy by association.

This view of 'trust' differs markedly from one endorsed by some bioethicists. Richard Zaner, for example, refers to the patient's trust in the physician as 'unavoidable.' He says, '[p]atients must trust not only physicians, but a host of other people as well, such as nurses, lab technicians, researchers'.[31] Zaner believes that patients trust their physicians because they 'have no choice but to trust'[32] and because professional trustworthiness is characteristic of every fiduciary relationship.[33] According to Pellegrino, '[we] are forced to trust professionals if we wish to have access to their knowledge and skill.'[34] He claims that trust is 'ineradicable.' He writes, '[t]o seek professional help is to trust that physicians possess the capacity to help and heal.'[35]

The problem with the no-choice-but-to-trust view is three-fold. First, there is empirical evidence, for example, that of Mechanic and Meyer, showing that patients are involved in a process of 'testing' their physicians' trustworthiness.[36] If trust were inevitable, patients would have no reason to test their physicians' trustworthiness. Second, there is evidence that trust in physicians, though persistent, is vulnerable, especially under some of the most aggressive versions of managed care.[37] Third, if the no-choice-but-to-trust view were true, it would seem to entail that at least some patients are the victims of widespread self-deception.

Many patients today are better informed and more active consumers of their medical care.[38] Studies show that patients are worried that their physicians don't spend enough time with them, that they won't make referrals, and that they compromise on the quality of care.[39] Other studies show that, although in general people give their health plans high ratings, they are concerned about managed care.[40] In view of this, it is difficult to see how some patients at least could both (1) hold the beliefs that they do about health care today and (2) continue to trust their physicians. To ascribe to patients both (1) and (2) would seem to commit them to believing something very close to a contradiction or to deny the validity of both the encapsulated interest and economic accounts of trust.

Perhaps some patients would be able to make the leap of faith necessary to hold contradictory beliefs. And some patients may believe that their physician will game the system.[41] But it is difficult to maintain that all, or even most, patients will continue to trust their physicians blindly in the face of as much contrary evidence as that to which patients are increasingly exposed in the media, for example. Of course, as we know from our discussion in Chapter 2 on the reluctance to make financial incentives transparent, there is certainly room for patient self-deception. Nonetheless, such self-deception, and the trust it breeds, is only as viable as the bluffing, puffing, and spinning that enables it.

There is empirical evidence that reimbursement mechanisms affect levels of trust. During the first half of 1997, Kao et al. found, in their study consisting of 2,086 telephone interviews, that the majority of patients trust their physicians regardless of payment method. Nonetheless, they also found somewhat lower levels of trust among patients in capitated systems than in fee-for-service.[42] This study also found that patients enrolled in fee-for-service were more likely to trust their health plans than those enrolled in managed care.[43] Another study found that choice of health plan could also influence trust.[44] Furthermore, there is evidence that cost containment mechanisms that limit physician autonomy, as many managed plans do, may adversely affect patient trust.[45] Sometimes the effect of managed care on patient trust can be indirect, by impairing continuity of care.[46] Later in this chapter, we will look at Mark Hall's view of trust, which treats trust in physicians as inevitable and largely immune to the contingencies of reimbursement schemes.

One last, but nonetheless important, point about trust is that it is a public good. As such, it carries with it the full moral force of other public goods. Public goods have two main characteristics: (1) non-rivalry in consumption and (2) non-excludability.[47] To say (1) that something is non-rivalrous in consumption is just to say that one person's use of it does not detract from another person's use. To say (2) that a good is non-excludable, is to say that we cannot easily exclude people from enjoying the benefits of the good.[48] Trust has both these characteristics. It is non-rivalrous in consumption insofar as one's ability to extend trust to one person is not limited by having already done so with another person. Trust is a non-excludable good because we cannot restrict the benefits of trust, such as social capital, to any particular people.

The doctor–patient relationship: a vessel of trust

The doctor–patient relationship with its long fiduciary history has been a relatively reliable and significant source of trust.[49] Physicians have the duty to act primarily in the interest of their patients, subordinating their own interests. Shielded by fiduciary duties, the doctor–patient relationship has been an important source of trust for both patients and the community. Early ethics codes encouraged physicians to carry themselves in ways that would cultivate trust.[50] No doubt such conduct was important at a time when physicians had little more to offer patients than comfort. Fiduciary duties created a context in which once in the 'hands of a physician,' patients could be assured of their impartial care.[51] More specifically, trust based on encapsulated interest could flourish with a relationship protected by fiduciary duties because fiduciary duties minimized the likelihood of conflicts of interest between patient and physician. It is also likely that trust within the doctor–patient relationship was reinforced because of its potential therapeutic benefits.[52]

Without trust, the interaction between doctor and patient would be significantly compromised.[53] Beginning at an early age, patients learned that their physicians would keep their secrets, act in their best interest, and, in the best of all possible doctor–patient relationships, exhibit care and concern for their welfare.[54] In order for physicians to make accurate and timely diagnoses, they must have adequate information from patients. Moreover, trust facilitates communication between patient and physician.[55] Safran and Taira found that patients who trust their physicians are more satisfied with their care.[56] Trust in physicians may also facilitate patient compliance with 'doctor's orders.'[57]

In the absence of a comparative study, common sense suggests that given the panoply of relationships we have, the doctor–patient relationship is a relatively important one from the perspective of producing trust. We are not at this point in a position to make any definitive assertions about how much trust and social capital the doctor–patient relationship is capable of producing. (This may have to do with the fact that trust and social capital are non-excludable public goods.) Nonetheless, it is still useful to consider how doctors score with respect to trust and to compare that with other professionals. According to a recent Gallup poll, 66 percent of Americans believe that doctors can be trusted.[58] The concept of trust used in the Gallup poll is different from the one that I have used. For each profession questioned, people were asked, '. . .tell me whether most of the people in [that profession] can be trusted or that you can't be too careful in dealing with them.'[59] Despite the conceptual difference, the question asked by the Gallup poll is compatible with the encapsulated interest account of trust and indeed may be operative in people's replies. As a profession, then, doctors fare well— though not as well as teachers at 84 percent, military officers at 73 percent, and police officers at 71 percent. Still, they have garnered more of the public's trust than accountants (51 percent), Catholic priests (43 percent), journalists (38 percent), stockbrokers (23 percent), and CEOs of large corporations (23 percent). (Finally, physicians have secured much more trust than the managers of HMOs, who only 20 percent of the American public believes can mostly be trusted.) Moreover, in July 2002, 41 percent of Americans believed that most people can be trusted. Although this may not seem high, the current level of trust is higher than it has been historically. According to the General Social Survey February 2000, 35 percent of the population said that they trusted most people. This improvement may be a result of the community coming together after 9/11.[60]

There are not many certain conclusions we can draw from these data. However, there are some interesting and fruitful speculations. First, given that overall trust levels are low and, according to the survey, especially low among the poorly educated (only 27 percent of those with a high school education or less believe that most people can be trusted), and given the importance of trust, it would be a mistake to remain passive with respect to relationships that foster trust. If anything, trust appears to be a relatively scarce resource.

Second, although physicians are by no means the most fruitful source of trust, garnering less trust than teachers, military and police officers, they nonetheless appear to be an important source of trust and perhaps are not easily duplicated. Physicians are likely to be encountered by everyone, and they may be a source of both thick and thin trust. Finally, if the less educated are less trusting in general, the doctor–patient relationship may be an important source of trust for them. Moreover, in view of the very low level of trust that Americans have in HMO managers, it is unlikely that they or their organizations can be counted on to provide trust as a substitute for the doctor–patient relationship.

As a community, we ought to be mindful of the possibility that as physicians come to be associated with HMOs, they may well find themselves less trusted.[61] There do not seem to be any strong reasons to think that the reverse will occur—that is, that the high trust for physicians will be transferred to MCOs. The fear is that in light of what we know about trust, and as the strategies of aggressively managed care become well known, physicians will be less trusted.

Medical trust at risk

Changes in how health care is delivered in this country compromise the ability of the doctor–patient relationship to continue to serve as a significant source of trust.[62] On the encapsulated-interest account, trust follows when the entruster can see that that it is in the interest of the trustee to be trustworthy. When patients can see that it is in their physicians' interest to be trustworthy, they will trust them.

Given increased patient familiarity with managed care, risk-sharing practices such as withholds, bonuses, and the unfortunate practice of cherry picking, compromised continuity of care, and the divided loyalties that ensue, it is unlikely, as a matter of logic, that patients could conclude that it is in the interest of their physicians to behave in ways that inspire trust. Physicians are clearly torn between their fiduciary duties to patients and some of their contractual obligations to health plans.[63] And although patients might take heart in the fact that their physicians are willing to lie to third-party payers on their behalf, they might also conclude, as a matter of logic and street epistemology, that if their physicians are willing to lie to others they will also lie, when push comes to shove, to patients.[64]

Trust that is based on a calculation of physician interests is at risk in managed-care plans because of the prevalence of conflicts of interest within managed care.[65] In an aggressively capitated system, for example, a physician may wind up in the midst of a conflict between a treatment decision and her own financial welfare.[66] Withholds and bonuses often amounting to a substantial portion of a physician's income can pit the physician's financial interest against the patient's health interest.[67] Moreover, shifting patient trust from physicians to organizations is not likely to be fruitful, in part, because trust in insurers is related to trust in physicians.[68] From the perspective of fostering patient trust based on encapsulated interest, organizations would seem to be worse off than physicians, since the loyalties of organizations are more narrowly focused than those of physicians. Although there are health plans that 'do well by doing good,' including some for-profit plans, for-profit health-care organizations primarily owe a duty of loyalty to shareholders, and patient care is a means to shareholder profits.[69] For-profit plans also have a very strong interest in courting payers/employers whose interests may not coincide with those patients. Indeed, MCOs refer to the money from premiums that are actually spent on health care as the 'medical loss ratio.' This language reflects the extent to which at least some MCOs are more 'profit-centered' than patient-centered.[70]

Physicians who work in managed care systems may have less interest in maintaining the good will of their patients. Capitation, for example, can challenge the physician's commitment to patient care and draw into question the assumption by patients that physicians can be counted on to put patients' interests first.[71] Patients may be required to change physicians when their own physician is dropped by the MCO or their employer drops the MCO. Kao and others have shown that managed-care reimbursement mechanisms adversely affect the level of trust that patients have for their physicians.[72] More recently, Gallagher et al. conducted a study in which 1,050 subjects were interviewed over the telephone about patient attitudes to bonuses given to physicians for controlling costs. Although 95 percent of respondents agreed that their physicians could be trusted to do what is best for their health, 60 percent of respondents said that a 10 percent cost control bonus would lower their trust in their doctor.[73] Thus patients themselves question the trustworthiness of physicians subject to aggressive managed-care incentives.

The economic or Bayesian approach to trust has two important implications for our understanding of trust within the doctor–patient relationship. First, it suggests that patients come to the doctor–patient relationship with different capacities for trust. They may be endowed with high levels of trust, plagued by low levels, or they may be somewhere in the middle. Physicians will have to adapt to these capacities. Nonetheless, as patients learn more about the current state of the health-care system through the media, friends, and personal experience, they are more likely to approach their physicians with distrust.[74] Second, the doctor–patient relationship has the potential to foster trust.[75] Today, however, instead of making a contribution to our 'trust fund,' this relationship is at risk of depleting it. Because subscribers are not fully knowledgeable of the incentives used by managed care, we can only begin to speculate about the extent to which their trust can be undermined.[76] The loss of trust in the face of strong need and high expectation may bring with it deeply felt disappointment.[77]

The risk is that eventually aggressive managed-care practices will alienate patients from their physicians and, in turn, continue to adversely affect levels of trust. A number of responses to this potential decline in trust are possible. Some responses would require changes to the funding arrangements that are at the heart of managed care. Others, however, involve changing our conception of trust and the possible role it will play in the traditional doctor–patient relationship. As we consider these responses, however, we need to be mindful not only of the implications for the doctor–patient relationship, but also for the community.

Coping with the problem of declining trust between doctor and patient

A trust-rich relationship between doctor and patient is replete with benefits most certainly for patients and perhaps also for physicians. Yet trust of this kind may well be incompatible with many of the cost containment mechanisms used by managed care, especially when they are aggressively implemented.[78] The tension between, on one hand, a trust-rich relationship and, on the other, aggressively managed medical care has led some ethicists to explore alternatives to trust. Thus far, two strategies stand out. In the first, trust in the doctor–patient relationship is replaced with trust in health-care organizations. In the second, the importance of preserving trust between doctor and patient is minimized because the assumption that trust is fragile is challenged.

Trust as procedural justice

Allen Buchanan's work on trust is illustrative of an approach that tries to cope with the threat of declining levels of trust in the doctor–patient relationship by shifting patient trust to the health-care organization itself.[79] Other authors have taken a similar tack.[80] Buchanan argues that there are two kinds of trust, 'status trust' and 'merit trust.' A person has status trust in virtue of inclusion in a profession that is regarded as trustworthy. In contrast, people possess merit trust because of abilities and behavior. When merit trust is primary, the physician is viewed as trustworthy because of her behavior. When merit trust is derivative, the organizations with which the physician is affiliated will be viewed as trustworthy.[81] He argues that within a managed-care context, we would be better off replacing the trust usually bestowed on physicians with trust based on the legitimacy of the organization. Buchanan believes that under managed care trustworthy organizations may help promote derivative merit trust. He advocates the following model. Trust ought to be based on the legitimacy of organizations which, in turn, should be based on the degree to which the organization: (1) reflects the core elements of procedural justice, (2) empowers employees and physicians to voice constructive criticism of organizational policies and identifies individuals to respond, and (3) recognizes a special responsibility of physicians to patients.[82]

The elements of procedural justice that would need to be present for an MCO to be legitimate are: (1) non-discrimination, (2) impartiality, (3) publicity of rules, (4) publicity of justifications for rules, and (5) accessible, fair, and timely procedures for appeals of denial of coverage. According to Buchanan, patients in an MCO do not have a justified interest in maximal care, but rather in having a legitimate organization.[83]

Thus, for Buchanan, the traditional fiduciary duty of physicians to put the interests of patients first is replaced with a conception of fair institutions. Buchanan defends this proposed transformation in the following way. First, he believes that a shift to procedural justice is warranted because no voice has authority with respect to health-care rationing in the United States. He argues that since it is close to impossible to pin down a definitive statement about what people are entitled to, we must find other ways of crafting just institutions. Buchanan believes that procedural justice is a good alternative.

Buchanan treats traditional medical ethics, or the fiduciary duty, as if it did little more than guide physicians to provide specific benefits. But fiduciary duties also serve as an important monitoring mechanism over physicians' inclinations to act opportunistically in their own interest.[84] It instructs physicians to put patients' interests first because patients are not well positioned to enforce their own interests.[85] Lest there be any doubt that some physicians would act opportunistically, recall the response of the medical community to the anthrax scare when a few physicians were found to be hoarding Cipro for themselves and their families.[86] Moreover, fiduciary duties in the medical profession have been instrumental in facilitating trust based on encapsulated interest by minimizing physician conflicts of interest. One has to wonder whether, in dismantling the fiduciary duties of physicians to patients, we may not be inadvertently encouraging opportunistic behavior by physicians or undermining an effective mechanism for trust. Before implementing such a change in the doctor–patient relationship, it would be prudent to ensure that all of the important benefits of the fiduciary duty can be met through other mechanisms, such as procedural justice.

Without the protective shield of fiduciary duties, and given the vulnerability of patients, physicians, like any one else, will seek their own best interests. Fiduciary duties provide a bright line, leaving little room for individual discretion about whose interests count. Even if we grant the advantages of procedural justice, the moral culture of many health care organizations is rooted in the ethics of shareholder primacy, which can put profit before patients.[87] As long as the primary interest of health plans lies with their shareholders, trust based on encapsulated interest will be difficult to come by in organizations.

It is also worth asking if what Buchanan describes as 'trust' qualifies as trust at all. On the face of it, trust based on the legitimacy of organizations strikes us as so different in depth and quality that it is unlikely to do the same work as trust in physicians. Within the doctor–patient relationship trust is the 'stuff' that facilitates the disclosure of private information that might in other contexts give rise to feelings of shame and embarrassment.

Buchanan justifies his endorsement of trust in the legitimacy of the organization on the grounds that there is no authoritative standard of substantive justice that can settle questions about health-care distribution. But is it really the case that there is no 'authoritative standard,' or is it rather the case that we are ignoring the various standards that exist? Within the U.S., the President's Commission determined that there is a 'right' to an adequate level of health care without undue burden.[88] It based this view on a number of factors, including the importance of health for equal opportunity within the U.S., the role of genetics in determining health, and the implications of poor health for everyone, not just the person who is ill. The American Medical Association supports the duty to provide materially beneficial care.[89] And the professional practice standard used in medical malpractice implies that all patients have a right to the same medical care.[90] From an international perspective, the World Health Organization enacted the Declaration of Alma Ata, requiring 'health for all.'[91] These standards have proclaimed that there is something akin to a right to health care.

Buchanan's conclusion that legitimate organizations are the best we can hope for under the circumstances is unwarranted. Moreover, he treats the trust between doctor and patient as a purely private matter, to be contracted away. But why assume that there is not a public dimension to trust? Once we take into account the social capital component of trust, the public's interest in trust cultivation should be acknowledged. If we acknowledge that trust has a morally important public dimension, then Buchanan would also need to show that (1) substituting procedural justice in place of substantive justice would not deplete existing levels of trust, and (2) trust understood as a legitimate organization has more to offer than trustworthy physicians in the traditional sense. I suspect that neither of these is true.

An organization's decision to deny health care that patients view as beneficial or life saving might be acknowledged by all concerned as legitimate, but nonetheless deplete status and merit trust. Finally, it would not be surprising if the very procedures needed to secure legitimacy, such as the review process and avenues for criticism of the institution, impaired the willingness and wherewithal of patients to trust. Consider the consequences of negotiating for medical care that one believes one needs in order to live or to save the life of a child. Trust based on encapsulated interest would be discouraged since the process itself would put the patient on notice about the possibility of conflicting interests. Negotiation may be especially regrettable because in some cases it would undermine trust unnecessarily. Review mechanisms might well require patients to negotiate for their health care, only to award them the benefits in the end. Throughout what is in essence an adversarial process, patients cum negotiators would lose trust in the physician and the organization, having reached an outcome better informed about conflicts of interest and trust weary from the process.[92] Moreover, the desire or need for a trust-rich, doctor–patient relationship will not go away.[93]

A procedural approach to ethics has also been endorsed by another group of ethicists. Randel and Pearson argue that many of the problems with which managed care is besieged should be understood as ethical problems and not as legal problems.[94] These ethicists have called their group BEST, which stands for 'Best ethical strategies for managed care.' Using this acronym, they refer to themselves at different times as the 'BEST team,'[95] the 'BEST approach,' or the 'BEST researchers.'[96] Although the acronym 'BEST' is amusing, it is also striking to see these persuasive techniques applied to 'ethics' itself.[97]

The BEST ethicists recommend that legal remedies be reframed in terms that look at the ethical performance of MCOs, but they suggest understanding ethics as 'a method of examining conflicts of values where there are competing interests, each of which represents a reasonable and justifiable position.'[98] They point out that a shift in how health care is delivered from patient-centered to a population-centered, capitated model has 'legitimately called into question the primacy of the central ethical value that previously prevailed in health care: the tradition of doing everything for the patient regardless of cost or degree of effectiveness.'[99] This seems to be a 'straw patient' argument. It has never been the case that *everything* was done for the patient regardless of cost. Under fee-for-service, fiduciary duties, mediated by the professional practice standard, guided physicians to put the interests of patients first and to consult with the community of physicians in determining what care to provide. But this is not the same as doing everything for the patient regardless of the cost. Moreover, the shift from patient-centered to population-centered is also somewhat of a fiction. In view of the fact that 63.5 percent of subscribers are enrolled in for-profit HMO plans (broadly understood), we might just as well characterize the shift as one from patient centered to shareholder-centered.[100] The decision about how much money to devote to patient care (medical loss ratio) is determined not only by the needs of the particular population of patients, but also by the demands of employers/payers, CEOs, and shareholders. As I suggested in Chapter 1, the fiduciary ethics of physicians to patients has not simply been called into question by a competing population ethic, but by a competing fiduciary ethic, namely, the fiduciary duty of managers and directors to shareholders.[101]

According to Randel and Pearson, a best practice is one that satisfies the following four criteria. (1) There is a coherent account of a problem, even if not identified as ethical, but embodying conflicting interests and falling within ten specific domains. (2) There is a plan of action to manage the ethical tension. This plan could be justified with reasons why the plan of action would achieve those ends. (3) There are systematically used procedures that would serve as effective ways to implement the plan. (4) There is a model to evaluate the effectiveness of the plan. Thus, according to the authors, 'best practices' are 'ethically noteworthy in that they engage diverse values, consider the various perspectives (the member, provider, and organization) and try to arrive at a reasonable policy that balances the views and values of all.'[102] Importantly, a best practice is one that has a structure that appears to ensure procedural fairness as opposed to substantive justice. Instead of providing, for example, adequate benefits, best ethical practices are ones that have the relevant subject matter (conflicts), are practical, follow procedures, and have some checks on effectiveness.

But what if the health interests of patients are morally more important than the interests of organizations and providers?[103] Although Buchanan endorses a procedural account of trust, he requires that legitimate organizations recognize the importance of patients. It might be argued that, because patients are more vulnerable and in greater need than are shareholders, they deserve greater concern and are entitled to special consideration. Spencer et al. argue, for example, that given the purpose of health-care organizations, patients are central.[104] We might also hold with good moral justification that the lives of patients are morally more important than the relatively high profits of shareholders.[105]

Purely procedural approaches of the kind endorsed by Randel and Pearson skirt the substantive issues. If the problems that surface in managed care have to do with how much of some good is distributed (denial of care), it is unlikely that they can be resolved through procedure. Underlying many of the acknowledged conflicts within managed care, such as the conflict of interest between patient and provider or provider and managed-care organization, are concerns about access to health-care resources. Consider the conflict between, on the one hand, the welfare of the patient and, on the other hand, the welfare of the health-care organization.[106] At issue is the interest of stockholders for profits and patients for medical care. The conflict that arises between patient and physician because of capitation is one about how to divide burdens and benefits between doctor and patient. From the fact that there is an impartial procedure in place for resolving the conflict, it does not follow that the needs of any one party are not more worthwhile morally than the other.

An approach that focuses on procedure misses the ethical point underlying disputes about substantive justice. Consider the occasions when procedural justice is adequate. John Rawls elucidated the idea of pure procedural justice by drawing an important distinction between perfect procedural justice and imperfect procedural justice. According to Rawls, perfect procedural justice occurs when there is an independent criterion for what is just and we are able to find a procedure that will achieve that just outcome. Having the child who cuts the cake take the last piece is an effective solution that will ensure the ideal outcome of an equal distribution.[107]

Imperfect procedural justice can be illustrated with the example of a trial. A fair outcome would be to have only a guilty defendant found guilty. A trial, with rules and evidence, is the procedure used to secure this outcome. Yet it cannot uniformly lead to the ideal outcome. It is imperfect. Gambling is an example of pure procedural justice. Here the outcome is fair simply because a fair process is followed. If a series of fair bets are made, any outcome is fair. The fair procedure ensures the fairness of the outcome because there is no independent criterion for a just outcome.[108]

Those who opt for a purely procedural conception of justice in health care treat health care as if it had no independent criterion of what a just outcome would be. They treat health care as if it were a lottery. Surely that is wrong. Although many people would disagree about what counts as justice in the distribution of health care, few would be willing to be identified with a view that treats health care like a lottery. Independently, we can determine that an ideal health-care distribution is one that would meet health-care needs (though we may certainly disagree about what constitutes a 'need'). Choosing a purely procedural approach here really commits one to maintaining the status quo.

Fragility of trust

Trust is precious. There is disagreement, however, about the fragility of trust and how best to promote it, whether through increased or decreased regulation.[109] Mark Hall develops the position that medical trust is more resilient than some scholars have assumed.[110] For this reason, he also challenges the assumption that increased regulation of managed care will promote trust. If trust is resilient, and if a 'hands off' approach is preferable to a 'hands on' approach, then the obligations we impute to organizations in order to ensure a large pool of trust would change.

Hall subscribes to the view that, although trust is important in a number of legal arenas, medical trust is unique. In particular, he claims that medical trust has a strong emotional basis.'[111] Hall states that at different times throughout the relatively recent history of health law, where one would have anticipated a decline in trust because of a change in the law, such a decline did not occur. For example, many people believed that confidentiality between doctor and patient was essential to preserving trust. They predicted that patient trust would diminish in the wake of *Tarasoff v. University of California*, a case that may be interpreted to have established a duty of physicians to violate patient confidentiality in order to warn third parties of imminent harm.[112] Yet a reduction in trust was not found by subsequent studies.[113] On the basis of this and similar phenomena, Hall concludes that trust 'may be more resilient than we often suppose, both in its ability to withstand various assaults, and in its glacial resistance to attempts to alter its course.[114] The moral of Hall's story is that patient trust is so resilient that we need not worry about assaults on it from managed care.

According to Hall, studies show that trust in physicians is systematically high and that patients continue to trust physicians. The qualities of physicians that facilitate trust seem to have to do with a physician's personality traits and relationship factors—for example, whether the physician is a good listener, exudes an air of confidence and whether the patient has chosen the physician and knows him well.[115] At the same time, he points out that although some of these same factors are present in institutions, overall trust in institutions is much lower than in individuals. The resilience of medical trust can be explained by the inevitability and need of patients to trust their physicians and to trust in the system of medicine. Patients trust physicians not only because of the individual traits of those physicians, but also because of a belief they have in the archetypal doctor.

Hall may be right, but another explanation can be given for why trust persists despite continuous assault on it. Both patients and physicians may be circumventing the implications of the assaults. Patients may trust physicians not because of an archetypal conception of the physician, but because they have some understanding of physicians' professional values and fiduciary duty. Patients may understand that physicians are first and foremost committed to their welfare. For example, an appeal in the Tarasoff case modified the duty to warn to a duty to protect. The latter gave physicians more latitude to find ways to alert third parties to potential harm or perhaps to hospitalize dangerous patients without violating confidentiality.[116] Thus far patient trust in physicians has remained relatively constant, not because of its inevitability but because, despite the presence of cost containment mechanisms that can impair trust, physicians motivated by their fiduciary duties have not yet permitted these incentives to interfere with the relationship between doctor and patient.[117]

Matthew Wynia's study showing that roughly 40 percent of physicians 'lie' to third-party payers to secure benefits for their patients, and that as many patients ask their physicians to lie for them, supports this conclusion.[118] In other words, it is reasonable to speculate that patients continue to trust their physicians (to the extent that they do) even in aggressively managed plans because those physicians are still putting the interests of patients first and, to some extent, not allowing managed care to erode trust.[119] Doctors and patients may in effect be colluding against managed care. What may appear to be the resilience of trust in the face of assault from managed care may in fact be the persistent refusal of some physicians to compromise their fiduciary duty to patients and to align themselves with MCOs.

Many physicians are trusted because they continue to behave in ways that patients typically associate with the trustworthiness of physicians— they show care and concern and continue to act as patient advocates. This behavior may allow patients to make certain inferences about physician interests. Although controversial, 'platinum' practices or 'boutique' practices are another way for physicians to have the kind of patient relationship that will facilitate high levels of trust. For an extra cost, patients receive more personalized attention from their physicians, including 24-hour telephone access, home visits, and the company of their physician to specialists.[120] Troyen Brennan suggests that luxury practices will allow physicians to devote more of their time to patient visits.[121] Dr Steven Flior, a Boston physician, explains why he started one of these practices, 'We want to be able to spend more time with patients. We are desperately struggling to create a system that lets us do that within the limitations of managed care.' His partner, Dr Bernard Karrinetsky, says, 'I couldn't stand it anymore—the day was an absolute treadmill. I wanted to devote more time to patients and I wanted to enjoy practicing.'[122] Although such practices have been criticized as unethical for abandoning patients, they are one of the ways and, as far as we know, a legal way for physicians to circumvent some of the adverse consequences of managed care reimbursement mechanisms.

Hall's argument that trust in physicians is primarily emotion based is also unconvincing. Much of the physician behavior that he identifies as associated with trust may also serve to reassure patients that their physicians do not have conflicting interests. Other behavior serves as the basis for reassuring patients of their physicians' universal commitment to patient welfare. In particular, some of the ways physicians comport themselves signal that they are committed to the principle of impartiality. Behavior, such as not discussing their personal lives, targets trust based on encapsulated interest by triggering certain patient beliefs, such as a belief in the selflessness of physicians.

Even if Hall were right that managed care has not thus far deeply impaired trust, it would be a mistake to assume that it will not do so in the future. Some studies have suggested that the public is unaware of how physicians are reimbursed.[123] Better-informed patients may be less willing to trust.[124] Other studies show that patients themselves believe that physicians who are under some economic influences are less trustworthy.[125] Still others show that trust has been impacted by reimbursement mechanisms.[126] One would anticipate that as continued pressure is placed on physicians to cut costs, especially in a poor economy, those who were once unwilling to comply with third-party imposed rationing will, in increasing numbers, conform to the standards of the new medicine. Moreover, since trust in institutions is low, the more physicians are identified with institutions as opposed to individuals, the less likely they are to be viewed as trustworthy.[127]

To substitute the rich trust between patient and physician with trust in institutions would be misguided. Trust in institutions may be a more diluted version of trust than what exists interpersonally. If I am right to view trust as a valuable resource, then it is wrong to exchange it at all, and especially wrong to exchange it for a less valuable form of trust. A more appropriate response would be for health-care organizations to look at the doctor–patient relationship as an important source of trust, better for health and for the community. From an economic perspective, money spent on maintaining a high-trust doctor–patient relationship may be money well spent. We should be cultivating both sources of trust.

Trust has become the proverbial 'hot topic.' From the amount of scholarship devoted to discussions of trust, including attempts to reconcile it with managed care, it is clear that few are content to let sleeping dogs lie. We have looked at two kinds of arguments against the view that trust in the doctor–patient relationship is important to preserve. In the first, it was suggested that we replace trust in the doctor–patient relationship with some form of trust founded in the procedural fairness of organizations. Second, we looked at the idea that trust is not as fragile as trust-based arguments that challenge managed care have assumed, and that therefore managed care is not the threat to trust that some have supposed. Both of these arguments attempt, in one way or another, to resolve the potential for trust-based problems in managed care by downplaying the significance of trust in the doctor–patient relationship.

A third option can also be identified, one that acknowledges the importance of trust for the doctor–patient relationship, but which treats it as vulnerable to assault. David Mechanic tries to strike a balance when he argues that though physicians are best suited to implement rationing, for the sake of trust, they may not be suited to inform patients of rationing decisions.[128] We looked at this question in the last chapter in our discussion of disclosure. Suffice it to say here that, given the relationship between truth, transparency, and trust, attempts to preserve trust by suppressing truth are at best paradoxical. Indeed, research on trust shows that trust is important and should be nurtured whenever possible.[129] Nonetheless, the most compelling *moral* argument in support of a doctor–patient relationship that enhances trust is to be found in a consideration of the benefits trust can bring to the community. In Chapters 4 and 5, we look at these benefits in our discussion of social capital.

Costs of conserving trust

Opting for a trust-rich doctor–patient relationship may undermine other values, such as liberty. Preserving trust in the way that I suggest may entail, for example, interfering with the liberty of organizations (MCOs to maximize the profits of shareholders or employers/payers to maintain their profit margins). Trust in physicians is based, as we have seen, on a number of factors, including the belief in physician competency and the belief that the physician will act in the patients' interests.[130] In some instances, maintaining trust may require acting against other interests of the community. Using Mill's harm principle Clancy and Brody argue, for example, that 'the physician who devotes expensive and marginally beneficial resources to the care of patient A might through the act be harming patients X, Y, and Z, who could have benefited much more substantially had these same resources been made available elsewhere.'[131] Of course, this argument is plausible in principle, but its persuasiveness hinges on the assumption that money that is not spent on patient A will be spent on patient B.

There is, however, no guarantee that within a health plan money not spent on one patient will be spent on other patients—perhaps especially not in the ever-expanding world of for-profit managed care. Moreover, given that the scarcity of medical resources is artificially imposed, there is similarly no reason to suppose that the 'original' amount allocated to health care (medical loss ratio) by payers and plans was adequate or just in the first place.[132] Indeed, during the first quarter of 2001, HMO earnings rose

8 percent from $298 million in the first quarter of 2000 to $322 in 2001. According to R. Weiss, this growth reflects the rate increases that HMOs imposed on consumers over the last three years.[133]

It is important to remember when invoking the harm principle, as Brody and Clancy do, that for Mill harm is a necessary, but not a sufficient condition for interfering with conduct.[134] For interference to be justified, it must also be the case that the interference will maximize overall the general happiness. Applied to health plans, the question is whether interfering with the relationship between doctor and patient and the physician's autonomy, in order to avoid harm to patients X, Y, and Z, causes too great a harm to the capacity for the relationship to produce trust. Thus, although we might grant for the sake of argument that in treating A we may harm X, Y, and Z, we may nonetheless create more harm by denying A marginally beneficial care, and the greater harm may be for all concerned. This would be so, for example, if denials of care resulted in much lower levels of trust and social capital. These lower levels of a valuable social good would potentially harm A, X, Y, and Z. By diminishing the trust between doctor and patient, we may, in turn, lose much of the richness of the relationship and its potential contribution to the community.

I have argued that trust between doctor and patient is an important social good. Efforts to compensate for the adverse impact of aggressively managed care on trust by substituting trust with legitimate organizations, with conflict resolution, or with optimism about medical trust's resilience, are unlikely to produce the trust-rich social benefits made possible by the doctor–patient relationship. In the next chapter, I develop the argument in support of the claim that trust between doctor and patient is good for the community.

Notes

1   A connection between truth/honesty and trust in doctors has been identified by D.H. Thom and B. Campbell. Patient–Physician Trust: An Exploratory Study. *Journal of Family Practice*, 1997; 44: 169–76; D. Mechanic and S. Meyer. Concepts of Trust Among Patients with Serious Illness. *Social Science and Medicine*, 2000; 51: 657–68; M.A. Hall et al. Trust in Physicians and Medical Institutions: What is it, Can it be Measured, and Does it Matter? *Milbank Quarterly*, 2001; 79: 613–39.
2   D.P. Sulmasy et al. Physicians' Ethical Beliefs About Cost-Control Arrangements. *Archives of Internal Medicine*, 2000; 160: 649–57; D. Mechanic and M. Schlesinger. The Impact of Managed Care on Patients' Trust in Medical Care and Their Physicians. *Journal of the American Medical Association*, 1996; 275: 1693–7; A.C. Kao et al. The Relationship Between Method of Physician Payment and Patient Trust. *Journal of the American Medical Association*, 1998; 280: 1708–14; see Hall et al., op. cit.; U.S.A. Today/CNN/Gallup Poll, 5–8 July 2002, as described in J.M. Jones. Poll Analyses: Americans Express Little Trust in CEOs of Large Corporations or Stockbrockers. *Gallup News Service*, 17 July 2002.
3   D. Mechanic. Changing Medical Organization and the Erosion of Trust. *Milbank Quarterly*, 1996; 74: 171–89; Hall et al., op. cit.

4 A. Buchanan. Trust in Managed Care Organizations. *Kennedy Institute of Ethics Journal*, 2000; 10: 209.

5 Kao et al. op. cit.

6 In a 2000 survey, the Kaiser Family Foundation found that, although most people are satisfied with their health plans, those in strictly managed plans were less satisfied than those in loosely managed plans. Kaiser Family Foundation. National Survey of Consumer Experiences with Health Plans: Survey of Finding and Chartpack, June 2000. According to a nationwide Harris Interactive Survey, 51 percent of respondents thought that managed care would harm the quality of medical care. Although this figure was down from 59 percent in 2000, the decline is attributed to the trend of managed care to manage more loosely. While Managed Care is Still Unpopular, Hostility Has Declined. H. Taylor and R. Leitman, eds. *Harris Interactive Health Care News* 2002; 2(5). Available at: http://harrisinteractive.com/news/letters_healthcare.asp.

7 E.H. Morreim. *Balancing Act: The New Medical Ethics of Medicine's New Economics*. Washington, DC: Georgetown University Press, 1995, 131; W.K. Mariner. Business v. Medical Ethics: Conflicting Standards for Managed Care. *Journal of Law, Medicine and Ethics*, 1995; 23: 240.

8 S. Dorr Goold. Money and Trust: Relationships between Patients, Physicians, and Health Plans. *Journal of Health Politics, Policy and Law*, 1998; 23: 689.

9 I suggest that it is fictional because very often the conditions for freely choosing a health plan do not exist. For example, many subscribers to a health plan are offered only one plan by their employers.

10 Mechanic, op. cit.

11 T. Bodenheimer. The American Healthcare System—the Movement for Improved Quality in Healthcare. *New England Journal of Medicine*, 1999; 340: 488–92.

12 Ibid.

13 Hall et al., op. cit.; Mechanic and Meyer, op. cit.

14 Ibid.; While Managed Care is Still Unpopular, Hostility Has Declined, op. cit.

15 Mechanic, op. cit.; B. Gray. Trust and Trustworthy Care in the Managed Care Era. *Health Affairs*, 1997; 16: 34–49; Mechanic and Schlesinger, op. cit., D. Mechanic. The Functions and Limitations of Trust in the Provision of Medical Care. *Journal of Health Politics, Policy and Law*, 1998; 23: 661–83; K. Grumbach et al. Resolving the Gatekeeper Conundrum. *Journal of the American Medical Association*, 1999; 282: 261–6.

16 Hall et al., op. cit.; Mechanic and Meyer, op. cit.; Buchanan, op. cit., pp. 189–212.

17 R. Hardin. Street-Level Epistemology of Trust. *Politics and Society*, 1993; 21: 506.

18 Ibid.

19 Ibid., p. 508.

20 Ibid., p. 507.

21 Ibid., p. 508.

22 Ibid.

23 R. Putnam. *Bowling Alone*. New York: Simon & Schuster, 2000, p. 136.

24 Mechanic, op. cit., p. 173.

25 P. Slovich. Perceived Risk, Trust and Democracy. *Risk Analysis*, 1993; 13: 677.

26 Mechanic and Meyer, op. cit.

27 Ibid.

28 Ibid.

29 Thom and Campbell, op. cit.

30 D.H. Thom. Physician behaviours that predict patient trust. *Journal of Family Practice* 2001; 50: 323–8.

31 R.M. Zaner. The Phenomenon of Trust and the Patient–Physician Relationship. In *Ethics, Trust, and the Professions: Philosophical and Cultural Aspects,* ed. E.D. Pellegrino et al. Washington, DC: Georgetown University Press, 1991, p. 49.

32 Ibid.

33 Ibid., p. 57.

34 E.D. Pellegrino. Trust and Distrust in Professional Ethics. In Pellegrino et al., *Ethics, Trust, and the Professions: Philosophical and Cultural Aspects,* op. cit., p. 69.

35 Ibid., p. 74.

36 Mechanic and Meyer, op. cit.

37 Mechanic, op. cit., p. 178; Kao et al., op. cit., p. 1713.

38 C.M. Cropper. The Take-Charge Patient: Now You and Your Physician Can Be Partners. That's Healthier for Everyone. *Business Week,* 26 August 2002; 3796: p. 154.

39 Kaiser Family Foundation. Consumer Views of the Impact of Managed Care. In *Trends and Indicators in the Changing Medical Marketplace,* 2002, Exhibit 7.5; A.A. Gawande et al. Does Dissatisfaction with Health Plans Stem from Having No Choices? *Health Affairs,* 1998; 17: 190; Kaiser Family Foundation/Harvard School of Public Health. National Survey on Consumer Experiences with and Attitudes Toward Health Plans. In *Trends and Indicators in the Changing Health Care Marketplace,* 2002, 82; R. Blendon et al. Understanding the Managed Care Backlash. *Health Affairs,* 1998; 17: 80–94.

40 Kaiser Family Foundation. National Survey of Consumer Experiences with Health Plans: Survey of Finding and Chartpack, op. cit.

41 M.K. Wynia et al. Physician Manipulation of Reimbursement Rules for Patients: Between a Rock and a Hard Place. *Journal of the American Medical Association,* 2000; 238: 1858–65. Patients who ask their physicians to lie to third-party payers for them would seem to both understand the 'mechanics' of managed care and trust their physicians.

42 Kao et al., op. cit.

43 Ibid.

44 A.C. Kao et al. Patients' Trust in their Physicians: Effects of Choice, Continuity, and Payment Method. *Journal of General Internal Medicine,* 1998; 13: 681–6.

45 K. Davis et al. Choice Matters: Enrollees' Views of Their Health Plans. *Health Affairs,* 1995; 14: 99–112.

46 D.P. Martin et al. Effect of a Gatekeeper Plan on Health Services Use and Changes: A Randomized Trial. *American Journal of Public Health,* 1989; 79: 1628–32; Kao et al. Patients' Trust in their Physicians: Effects of Choice, Continuity, and Payment Method, op. cit.

47 I. Kaul et al. (eds). *Global Public Goods.* New York: Oxford University Press, 1999, p. 3.

48 Ibid., p. 4

49 M. Rodwin. *Medicine, Money & Morals: Physicians' Conflicts of Interest.* New York: Oxford University Press, 1993, pp. 183–4; E.D. Pellegrino, op. cit., p. 72; Zaner, op. cit., p. 45; F. Fukuyama. *Trust: The Social Virtues and the Creation of Prosperity.* New York: The Free Press, 1995, p. 19; M. Hall. Trust, Law and Medicine. *Stanford Law Review,* 2002; 55: 463–527; Mechanic, The Functions and Limitations of Trust in the Provision of Medical Care, op. cit.

50 Hippocratic Corpus, The Physician, Decorum, XVI.

51 This is not to say that where there are fiduciary duties, there are no bad nor greedy physicians. Certainly, widespread practices such as Medicaid mills and 'patient dumping', both of which preceded managed care, suggest that greedi-

ness can accompany fiduciary duties. Still, it is likely that fiduciary duties limit this conduct in a way that the principle of *caveat emptor* would not.

52 A.K. Shapiro and E. Shapiro. Patient–Provider Relationships and the Placebo Effect. In *Behavioral Health*, ed. J.D. Matarazzo et al. New York: J. Wiley and Sons, 1984, p. 378.

53 S. Greenfield et al. Patients' Participation in Medical Care: Effects on Blood Sugar Control and Quality of Life in Diabetes. *Journal of General Internal Medicine*, 1988; 3: 448–57; S. Greenfield et al. Expanding Patient Involvement in Care: Effects on Patient Outcomes. *Annals of Internal Medicine*, 1985; 102: 520–8; S.H. Kaplan et al. Assessing the Effects of Physician–Patient Interaction on the Outcomes of Chronic Disease. *Medical Care*, 1989; 27(suppl): S5110–27.

54 Mechanic, Changing Medical Organization and the Erosion of Trust, op. cit.

55 D. Roter and J. Hall. *Doctors Talking with Patients/Patients Talking with Doctors: Improving Communication in Medical Visits*. Westport, CT: Auburn House, 1992.

56 D.G. Safran and D.A. Taira. Linking Primary Care Performance to Outcomes of Care. *Journal of Family Practice*, 1998; 47: 213–20.

57 R.A. Scott and L. Aiken. Organizational Aspects of Caring. *Milbank Quarterly*, 1995; 73: 77–95; B.H. Gray. Trust and Trustworthy Care in the Managed Care Era. *Health Affairs*, 1997; 16: 34–49.

58 U.S.A. Today/CNN/Gallup Poll, op. cit.

59 M. Strausberg, e-mail message to Data Librarian of Gallup Poll, 13 September 2004; see also Jones, op. cit.

60 R. Putnam. *Bowling Alone*. New York: Simon & Schuster, 2000.

61 Mechanic and Schlesinger, op. cit.

62 Mechanic, Changing Medical Organization and the Erosion of Trust, op. cit.

63 See, for example, M. Angell. Medicine: The Endangered Patient-Centered Ethic. *Hastings Center Report*, February 1987; S. Shortell et al. Physicians as Double Agents: Maintaining Trust in an Era of Multiple Accountabilities. *Journal of the American Medical Association*, 1998; 280: 1102–8; E.J. Emanuel and N. Neveloff Dubler. Preserving the Physician–Patient Relationship in the Era of Managed Care. *Journal of the American Medical Association*, 1995, 273: 323–9.

64 Wynia et al., op. cit., p. 1861.

65 M. Rodwin. *Medicine, Money & Morals: Physicians' Conflicts of Interest*. New York: Oxford University Press, 1993, p. 180.

66 M.E. Sorbero et al. The Effect of Capitation on Switching Primary Care Physicians. *HSR: Health Services Research*, Vol. 38, Part 1, 2003; Rodwin, op. cit.

67 Dorr Goold, op. cit., pp. 687–95.

68 Mechanic and Schlesinger, op. cit.; see also B. Zheng et al. Development of a Scale to Measure Patients' Trust in Health Insurers. *Health Services Research*, 2002; 37: 187–202.

69 *Dodge v. Ford Motor Co.*, 204 Mich. 459, 170 N.W. 668 1919; Revised Model Business Code 858.30(a)(1992); Revised Model Business Code 4.01 (9c). For an argument against this view, see P. Illingworth. A Role for Stakeholder Ethics in Meeting the Ethical Challenges Posed by Managed Care Organizations. *HEC Forum*, 1999; 11: 306–22.

70 T. Bodenheimer. The HMO Backlash—Righteous or Reactionary. *New England Journal of Medicine*, 1996; 335: 160; J.P. Kassirer. The New Health Care Game. *New England Journal of Medicine*, 1996; 335: 433.

71 F. Chervenak et al. Responding to the Ethical Challenges Posed by the Business Tools of Managed Care in the Practice of Obstetrics and Gynecology. *American Journal of Obstetrics and Gynecology*, 1996; 175: 523–7.

72 Kao et al. The Relationship Between Method of Physician Payment and Patient Trust, op. cit., p. 1712. For another view, see M.A. Hall et al. How Disclosing HMO Physician Incentives Affects Trust. *Health Affairs*, 2002; 21: 197–206.

73 T.H. Gallagher et al. Patients' Attitudes Toward Cost Control Bonuses for Managed Care Physicians. *Health Affairs*, 2001; 20: 189.

74 D. Mechanic, Changing Medical Organization and the Erosion of Trust, op. cit., p. 177.

75 U.S.A. Today/CNN/Gallup Poll, op. cit. This follows given the traditional high trust quality of the relationship, especially when compared to other sources of trust.

76 P.J. Cunningham et al. Do Consumers Know How Their Health Plans Work? *Health Affairs*, 2001; 20: 159–66; Hall et al., How Disclosing HMO Physician Incentives Affects Trust, op. cit.; S.L. Issaacs. Consumers' Information Needs: Results of a National Survey. *Health Affairs*, 1996; 15: 31–41; T.E. Miller and C.R. Horowitz. Disclosing Doctors' Incentives: Will Consumers Understand and Value the Information? *Health Affairs*, 2000; 19: 149–55.

77 Zaner, op. cit.; Kao et al. for example, found a correlation between trust and health. That is, healthier patients seemed to be more willing to trust their physicians. The converse may also be true, and the sicker the patients are, the less willing they are to trust their physicians. Further research should be done on this question. Kao et al. The Relationship Between Method of Physician Payment and Patient Trust, op. cit.

78 Ibid.; Mechanic, Changing Medical Organization and the Erosion of Trust, op. cit.

79 A. Buchanan. Trust in Managed Care Organizations. *Kennedy Institute of Ethics Journal*, 2000; 10: 209.

80 D. Mechanic. Managed Care and the Imperative for a New Professional Ethic. *Health Affairs*, 2000; 19: 100–12.

81 Buchanan, op. cit., p. 191.

82 Ibid., pp. 195–6.

83 Ibid., p. 204.

84 R.C. Clarke. Agency Costs versus Fiduciary Duties. In *Principles and Agents: The Structure of Business*, ed. J.W. Pratt and R.J. Zeckhauser. Boston: Harvard Business School Press, 1985, p. 73.

85 Ibid., p. 74.

86 Personal communication with physicians.

87 Mariner, op. cit., 241.

88 President's Commission for the Study of Ethical Problems in Medicine and Biomedical and Behavioral Research. Securing Access to Health Care. From *Securing Access to Health Care*. Vol. 1 (U.S. Government Printing Office, 1983). In: *Contemporary Issues in Bioethics*, 5th ed, ed. T.L. Beauchamp and L. Walters. Belmont, CA: Wadsworth Publishing Company, 1999, pp. 362–8.

89 The American Medical Association Council on Ethical and Judicial Affairs, Code of Medical Ethics Current Opinions and Annotations 8.13 (2)(b). Chicago: AMA, 2002–2003, p. 219.

90 *Davis v. Virginia RR Co.* 361 U.S. 354, 357, 1960; see W. Prosser & W. Keeton. *Prosser and Keltor on the Law of Torts*, 5th ed. St. Paul, Minn.: West Publishing Company, 1984, pp. 164–5.

91 Declaration of Alma Ata. International Conference on Primary Health Care, Alma-Ata, U.S.S.R., 6–12 September 1978.

92 A.I. Applbaum. *Ethics for Adversaries*. Princeton: Princeton University Press, 1999, p. 48.

93 To meet this need, we may find ourselves saddled with a two-tiered system in which wealthy patients purchase insurance that provides them with a fiduciary doctor and the poor, or inadequately insured, simply settle for a legitimate organization. Two Boston internists, for example, announced that for an annual fee of $4,000 per patient, they would provide a more personalized form of medical care. These new so-called 'platinum practices' provide patients who can afford them with the benefits of a high-trust, 'doctor as fiduciary' relationship.

94 L. Randal et al. How Managed Care Can Be Ethical. *Health Affairs*, 2000; 20: 43–56.

95 Ibid.

96 Ibid.

97 Ibid.

98 Ibid.

99 Ibid.

100 Kaiser Family Foundation. *Chartbook: Trends and Indicators in the Changing Health Care Marketplace*, May 2002.

101 W.K. Mariner. Rationing Health Care and the Need for Credible Scarcity: Why Americans Can't Say No. *American Journal of Public Health*, 1995; 85: 1439–45; P. Illingworth. A Role for Stakeholder Ethics in Meeting the Ethical Challenges Posed by Managed-Care Organizations. *HEC Forum*, 1999; 11: 306–22.

102 Randal et al., op. cit., p. 51.

103 E. Spencer et al. (eds). *Organizational Ethics in Healthcare*. New York: Oxford University Press, 2000, p. 62; see also K.T. Christensen. Ethically Important Distinctions Among Managed Care Organizations. *Journal of Law, Medicine and Ethics*, 1995; 23: 223–9.

104 Spencer et al., op. cit.; Illingworth, op. cit., p. 308.

105 For an argument supporting this conclusion and others similar to it, see P. Singer. Famine, Affluence, and Mortality, and the Single Solution to World Poverty. In *Writings on an Ethical Life*. New York: HarperCollins, 2000.

106 Illingworth, op. cit., p. 310; W.K. Mariner. Business vs. Medical Ethics: Conflicting Standards for Managed Care. *Journal of Law, Medicine and Ethics*, 1995; 23: 238.

107 J. Rawls. Distributive Justice. In *J. Rawls Collected Papers*, ed. S. Freeman. Cambridge, MA: Harvard University Press, 1967, p. 148.

108 Ibid., p. 149.

109 For arguments in support of the fragility of trust, see, for example, B. Barber. *The Logic and Limits of Trust*. New Brunswick, NJ: Rutgers University Press, 1983; P. Slovick. Perceived Risk, Trust and Democracy. *Risk Analysis*, 1993; 13: 675–82.

110 Hall, op. cit.

111 Ibid.

112 *Tarasoff v. Regents of the University of California*, 1974. Sup. 118 Cal. Rptr. 129.

113 A.A. Stone. Paradigms, Pre-emptions, and Stages: Understanding the Transformation of American Psychiatry by Managed Care. *International Journal of Law and Psychiatry*, 1995, 18: 353–87.

114 Hall, op. cit.

115 Ibid.

116 L.R. Wulsin et al. Unexpected Clinical Features of the Tarasoff Decision: the Therapeutic Alliance and the 'Duty to Warn'. *American Journal of Psychiatry*, 1983; 140: pp. 601–3.

117 Pellegrino, op. cit., p. 72.
118 Wynia et al., op. cit.
119 M. Gregg Bloche. Fidelity and Deceit at the Bedside. *Journal of the American Medical Association*, 2000; 283: 1881–3.
120 P. Belluck. Doctors' New Practices Offer Deluxe Service for Deluxe Fee. *New York Times*, 15 January 2002, Sec. A1.
121 T. Brennan. Luxury Primary Care—Market Innovation or Threat to Access? *New England Journal of Medicine*, 2002; 346: 1165–8.
122 Belluck, op. cit.
123 Kao et al., The Relationship Between Method of Physician Payment and Patient Trust, op. cit.; Miller and Horowitz, op. cit.
124 D. Mechanic. Dilemmas in Rationing Health Care Services: The Case for Implicit Rationing. *British Medical Journal*, 1995; 310: 1655–9; D. Mechanic. Models of Rationing: Professional Judgment and the Rationing of Medical Care, 140 *University of Pennsylvania Law Review* 1713, May 1992.
125 Gallagher et al., op. cit., p. 189.
126 Mechanic, Changing Medical Organization and the Erosion of Trust, op. cit.
127 R. Blendon et al. Understanding the Managed Care Backlash. *Health Affairs*, 1998; 17: 80–110.
128 Mechanic, Dilemmas in Rationing Health Care Services: The Case for Implicit Rationing, op. cit.; Mechanic, Models of Rationing: Professional Judgment and the Rationing of Medical Care, op. cit.
129 Evidence for this is extensive and diverse. F. Fukuyama. *Trust: The Social Virtues and the Creation of Prosperity.* New York: The Free Press, 1995; Putnam, op. cit.; G. Brenkert. Trust, Morality, and International Business. *Business Ethics Quarterly*, 1998; 8: 293–317; N. Kumar. The Power of Trust in Manufacturer–Retailer Relationships. *Harvard Business Review*, November 1996, pp. 92–106; R. La Porta et al. Trust in Large Organizations. *AEA Papers and Proceedings*, 1997; 87: 333–8; Mechanic and Meyer, op. cit.
130 Ibid.
131 C.M. Clancy and H. Brody. Managed Care: Jekyll or Hyde? *Journal of the American Medical Association*, 1995; 273: 338–9.
132 W. Mariner. Rationing Health Care and the Need for Credible Scarcity: Why Americans Can't Say No, op. cit.
133 R. Weiss. HMO Earnings Climb to $322 Million in First Quarter 2001. *Business Wire*, 26 November 2001.
134 See J.S. Mill. *On Liberty.* Cambridge: Hackett Publishing Company, 1978, p. 9.

4 The doctor–patient relationship in a social context

In 1996, a three-month-old girl was taken to the pediatric oncology group at the University of North Carolina Hospital. After she was diagnosed with leukemia, her physician recommended a bone marrow transplant. There were two excellent transplant facilities nearby. Nonetheless, the family's HMO asked the physicians to refer the baby to what it called a 'center of quality,' a transplantation center in another state that the HMO had approved for that region.

The baby's physicians were not concerned about the quality of care she would receive at the new center, but they were concerned about the emotional hardship on the family should they have to leave the state for several months in order to have the baby cared for. Employment considerations meant that the baby's father would not be able to join his family. For the mother to accompany her baby, she would have to give up her job, take a pay cut, or be demoted to a job of lesser status. The baby's older sister, who was already experiencing behavior problems, would now have to be separated from her mother. Furthermore, the family would be placed under financial duress as they tried to negotiate a temporary relocation to another state. It perhaps goes without saying that such a relocation would also take them away from extended family, friends, and the other support networks on which they had come to rely. The baby's physicians asked the HMO to refer the baby to a closer facility, but the HMO refused and accused the physicians of interfering with the 'client–carrier relationship.'[1]

The baby received the bone marrow transplant out-of-state and tolerated it well. In the process, the baby's mother was demoted, her father lost his job, and the older daughter had to live with relatives out of state. These problems were exacerbated when, after experiencing a relapse, the baby was sent to yet another transplantation center. The first center was no longer regarded by the HMO as a 'center of quality.'

When the story of this family's experience appeared in the *New York Times*, not surprisingly it captured the attention of readers.[2] People sympathized with the plight of the family. Not only did they have to face the prospect of losing a child, but they had to confront it away from home and without the support of their community, friends, family, and colleagues. It is difficult for most of us to imagine the former, let alone the latter. This case illustrates how some cost containment strategies can put our reservoir of trust and social capital at risk. By separating the family from its social network, the HMO deprived the family of the trust and social capital it had cultivated, leaving it to cope without access to these resources. Because trust and social capital are enriched by successful trust-based interactions, an opportunity to further enhance the reservoir was lost.

Regrettably, experiences similar to those of this family are not uncommon in today's health-care climate, where patient-centered care is gradually being replaced with the ethic of the marketplace.[3] Although the family's HMO provided the baby with the needed bone marrow transplant, by fragmenting care it deprived the baby and family of the social resources the family had developed over the years, resources to help them cope with just such an ordeal. In so doing, it put the health of the baby and the family at greater risk.[4]

In Chapter 3, I argued that the doctor–patient relationship is an important source of trust, and that some managed-care cost containment mechanisms have put trust from this source at risk.[5] Trust in the doctor–patient relationship also has advantages for the community. In this chapter and the next, I shall discuss these. Scholars from a number of fields, including sociology and public health, have studied the health benefits conferred on people when they have an extensive web of social relations and relative equality within them. Recently, ethicists have begun to integrate these approaches into bioethics discussions.[6] When the doctor–patient relationship is viewed in a social context, we can more easily see how it might contribute to the overall welfare of the community.

To this end, I look at three dimensions of the doctor–patient relationship: (1) its potential as a relationship that promotes the health of the individual and the community, and (2) the potential benefits it can produce when it reflects principles of equality. In Chapter 5, I look at (3) the doctor–patient relationship as a source of social capital. I argue that once we take into account the social dimensions of the doctor–patient relationship, it is difficult to tolerate the burdens that some aggressive versions of managed care impose on the community.[7] I divide this discussion into two chapters because the analysis of (3), social capital, includes a moral argument that, though relevant to (1) and (2), is most directly relevant to (3). Regrettably, there have been few empirical studies of the social consequences of reimbursement mechanisms. My hope is that identifying the moral issues will help to generate such studies.

Social relations are important for health promotion

Looking at the doctor–patient relationship in a social context reveals its capacity to contribute to the community. The recent studies of social epidemiologists show that[8] the degree to which people are embedded in a web of social relationships that provide intimacy, love and meaning as well as a larger sense of belonging and 'fit' with a larger community will have positive effects on their health. In particular, social relations have been shown to: (1) influence health outcomes across the life course and (2) influence disease prevalence, progression, mortality, and physical and cognitive functions.

Positive social relationships are good for your health. Relationships with spouse and partner, family, friends, colleagues, and voluntary and religious organizations seem to be health promoting.[9] Studies show that the more extensively people are integrated into a social web, the better their health is likely to be.[10] Although not yet the focus of a study, one would expect that the relationship between doctor and patient is among those relationships that are health-promoting for people. It promotes health directly through delivery of health care, but also indirectly as a mechanism of social support.

Studies have found that communities abundant in social cohesion are health promoting.[11] People in the small town of Roseto, Pennsylvania, were studied extensively and, despite similar risk factors for smoking, obesity, and fat intake, were found to have half the death rate from heart attacks as those living in neighboring towns.[12] These studies concluded that their good health was a result of the close-knit social relationships in Roseto, or 'social cohesiveness.' Durkheim defines 'social cohesiveness' as a society in which there is plenty of 'mutual moral support, which instead of throwing the individual on his own resources, leads him to share in the collective energy and supports his own when exhausted.'[13] According to Kawachi and Berkman, cohesiveness is a subset of social capital.[14] Because the doctor–patient relationship focuses on the care and healing of patients, it reflects some of the values of support and concern that are at the heart of social cohesion.[15] Trust may be an essential ingredient of social cohesion as it is of social capital. Conceptually, it is difficult to imagine that moral support could be effective in the absence of trust. Certainly the fact that the social survey showed that 66 percent of Americans trust their physicians bodes well for the healing relationship as a source of trust, social cohesion, and social capital.[16]

An overview of some of the studies of social epidemiologists will be helpful. According to Lisa Berkman, Director of the Center for Social Epidemiology at Harvard School of Public Health, people who are isolated are at greater risk of early death than people who are socially integrated.[17] In one study, Berkman and others found that people in Alameda County who lacked social ties were 1.9 to 3.1 times more likely to die in the nine-year follow-up period.[18] According to Berkman, people who die early because of a lack of social connectedness are dying from ischemic heart disease, cerebrovascular and circulatory disease, cancer, and respiratory and gastrointestinal illnesses.[19] Moreover, the correlation between social isolation and risk of early death was independent of high-risk behavior such as smoking and alcohol consumption. Another study of social connectedness conducted in Durham County compared measures of (1) self-perceived social support (loneliness), (2) impaired social roles and attachments, and (3) low frequency of social interaction. This study showed that people who were lonely, had impaired social relations, or infrequent social interactions are at greater risk of dying earlier than others.[20]

Studies that examine the effect of social relations on specific conditions also confirm the findings of this research. Hoffman and Hatch found that social support of the mother by a family member improved fetal growth.[21] People who are recovering from a heart attack have been shown to benefit from social ties, especially the social support provided by intimate ties.[22] A Swedish study of 150 cardiac heart patients found that patients who were socially isolated had three times the ten-year mortality rate of those who were socially integrated.[23]

Several explanations for why social relations are important for health have been offered. According to Berkman, social networks might be important because they enhance accessibility to health care. Second, social networks might be key to certain socio-environmental conditions. Third, social networks and easy access to social support may increase the presence of health-promoting behavior. The Alameda County study, for example, showed that people who lack social ties tend to have more unhealthy behavior, such as smoking and alcohol consumption.[24] Perhaps smokers and drinkers are trying to comfort themselves in the face of feelings of loneliness. Social isolation may create a chronically stressful condition that results in the body aging at a faster pace.[25]

Studies of this kind are morally significant because they underscore the existence of a harm and presumably an avoidable harm. People without extensive social relations appear to be harmed by the absence of these contacts. When people are deprived of social relations, either directly (because a spouse dies) or indirectly (social arrangements that alienate people from each other), they are thereby harmed. Naturally, consequentialists will want to avoid such harms. From a bioethics perspective the data from social epidemiologists are important because they show that impoverished social relations put people's health at risk. Ultimately, bioethics is interested in the health of individuals, and in ensuring that caretaking occurs in an ethical manner.[26] From the perspective of understanding the importance of the doctor–patient relationship as a source of trust, this research should not be ignored.

Ideally, having acknowledged the importance of social relations, health policy can be crafted to create and foster social relations among community members. The public policy that we implement can help people develop their ability to value, share, and sustain social relations. Berkman recommends that policy makers be mindful of the following four factors:

(1) Evidence suggests that both intimate and extended relationships that originate in voluntary and religious affiliations are important and health promoting.
(2) Social networks originate in diverse relationships. Today's families come in a variety of shapes and sizes. Policies that respect this panoply of relationships will be health promoting.
(3) Social support also comes from a variety of sources. It is important to be open-minded about who provides support.
(4) Social networks are ever changing and are influenced by learned ability, and social and economic factors.[27]

Public policy has the capacity to facilitate family and community relationships in a number of ways. For example, corporate policies that recommend moving employees around at critical times of family development compromise important social relations.[28] Policies that encourage family-friendly workplaces and parental leave also will be health-promoting. Indeed, policies and laws that promote family and friendship would seem preferable, from this standpoint, to those that do the opposite.

Similar considerations can be applied to our health-care system. It can either promote or undermine the creation of social networks. The relationships among physicians, other providers, and their patients are important in this respect. At their best, providers deliver not only competent clinical care, but also emotional support to vulnerable patients.[29] In many ways, these relationships are paradigmatic of supportive relationships. Nurses, for example, spend an enormous amount of time with patients, especially in hospital settings. The American Nursing Association identifies the following activities as constituting the practise of nursing: (1) attention to the full range of human responses to health and illness; (2) the integration of objective data with subjective data gained from the patient's experience; (3) the application of scientific knowledge to diagnosis and treatment; and (4) 'the provision of a caring relationship.'[30] Given the nursing focus on individual patient care, the expression of care and concern, and their connection to trust, quality nursing care is important for social capital. Physicians are also well positioned to either make patients feel deeply cared for as part of a healing community, or to exacerbate their feelings of loneliness and alienation by cultivating the opposite feelings.

Fragmenting patient care by requiring patients to travel to remote locations for tests and procedures takes them away not only from familiar clinicians, but also from loved ones and other social networks at a time when they are in need of close ties. This was the case for the North Carolina family that was described at the beginning of this chapter. It would not be surprising if, in the case of very sick patients or those with chronic illnesses, much of their social interaction is with people from within the medical system. Either they will be able to draw on the health-care system for needed support or, at the worst, will face an impoverished doctor–patient relationship and be taken away from the support of their local community.

Reimbursement mechanisms that create the context for physicians to prefer healthy patients over sick ones, or to spend less time with patients, or require patients to change physicians, or that interfere with the relationship between doctor and patient in other significant ways impair the potential of the relationship to promote health. The presence of intermediaries, such as utilization review and gatekeeper practices, can also disrupt the potential benefits from the doctor–patient relationship.[31] Moreover, economic incentives that encourage doctors to see their own financial interests as at odds with the interests of their patients place a strain on the relationship between patient and physician.[32] Given what we know about health-promoting relationships, the potential of the doctor–patient relationship to promote health would change with the quality of that relationship. Under aggressively implemented managed care, patients and their communities are deprived of some of the benefits of the doctor–patient relationship.[33] And insofar as aggressively managed care removes a much-needed support from patients, it puts the health of patients at risk.

Cost containment mechanisms such as capitation and attending strategies such as cherry picking (choosing to see healthy patients) have the effect of pitting physician against patient.[34] Cost containment mechanisms that limit access to specialists will have adverse outcomes for patients with chronic conditions.[35] Patients, in turn, may have an incentive to deceive their physicians about their health or to shop for more resource-friendly doctors. Both of these may well discourage a trust-rich relationship between doctor and patient. But there are other social relationships indirectly connected with doctor–patient relationships that may also suffer.

As patients become more knowledgeable of the financial arrangements within health plans, and as it becomes more difficult for them to access resources, we may find them competing with each other for medical resources as they now compete to access scarce organs or clinical trials. Although there were no studies on this at the time of writing, such competition among patients makes sense under the circumstances. Mindful of scarcity and with less trust available, patients may be less content to wait their turn. As patients become aware of the so-called 'duty of stewardship' (the duty of physicians to protect resources for the community), and as they realize that they may not receive care because others will receive it, they may view fellow patients as competitors for these prized resources. Thus, patient–patient relationships may be compromised by the health-care system. Instead of being able to provide support to each other as members of support groups, patients may try to edge out fellow patients. By underscoring the competitive relationships among patients for resources, managed care may undermine the benefits to be had from the primary relationship between doctor and patient, as well as from secondary relationships that are indirectly dependent on it—such as those formed within a support group. Given the importance of social relations for health, this is one area deserving of further research.

As of now many of the cost containment mechanisms used by MCOs remain veiled from patients.[36] Moreover, requiring patients to change doctors as frequently as they may change jobs can undermine trust between doctor and patient and thereby separate patients from health-promoting social ties.[37] Cost containment mechanisms that target physician behavior, when practiced transparently, are likely to diminish trust and social capital within a particular community of patients.[38] If attempts are made to obscure incentives from patients, they may be unsuccessful or even backfire with respect to trust.

Given the importance of social relations for health, it would seem contrary to patient welfare to compromise these relationships.[39] It is also worth speculating that since MCOs engage in extensive cost shifting (e.g., sending patients home to recuperate from surgery), it is especially important for them to maintain high levels of trust and social capital. For example, health plans may reduce hospital stays, forcing patients to rely more heavily on social support systems. Yet, they undermine the wherewithal of patients to rely on those networks. This seems counterproductive at best.

The impact of income inequality on health

A connection between low income and poor health has been widely acknowledged.[40] It may be that the wealthy and middle class have access to many of the ingredients of health, including better food, better living conditions, and better education, which, in turn, give them improved access to information. Alternatively, the advantages of better education may confer improved social status, which, in turn, benefits health.[41] There is also evidence that reducing economic disparity above a certain level of income is good for health.[42]

For a variety of reasons, including the need to make sense of the fact that the richest countries in the world do not necessarily have the healthiest populations, many scholars have speculated that what makes the difference is not absolute income, or whether a person is rich or poor, but above a certain level relative income.[43] According to the relativist, it is not simply low income or poverty per se, but rather the presence of income inequality that puts health at risk. Studies have shown that more egalitarian communities tend to have healthier populations.[44] If the relativist's position is correct, then, some have argued, we might well have greater success improving health outcomes, not by pouring more money into health care, but by improving people's lives overall and diminishing social gaps.

Although it is not clear why social status would negatively affect health, Wilkinson speculates that it may have to do with the biology of chronic anxiety.[45] Studies on nonhuman primates support this as well. One study of macaques in captivity showed a direct link between low social status and increased arteriosclerosis, obesity, and higher cortisol levels.[46] Worrying over long periods of time can take a physical toll on individuals.

It is certainly plausible that social status has an impact on health and at least partially because of anxiety. Although a concern to keep up with the Joneses might have its rewards, clearly a disadvantage is the anxiety created by the often-frustrated wish to keep up. Subsequent studies, including those that take into account Whitehall II (a study of British civil servants measuring the relationship between social class/employment rank and health status),[47] show that the degree of control one has at work can affect health outcomes.[48] According to this explanation, social inequalities are thought to mirror differences in control over work. Again, as with connectedness and social relations, there is good evidence that 'control' has a positive impact on overall happiness levels. In studies done by psychologists, autonomy, defined as the feeling that your activities are self-endorsed and self-chosen, was fundamental for happiness.[49] These studies support the results of the second Whitehall study that 'control' is behind the differences we see underlying social inequality.

Managed care and the erosion of the professional practice standard

Health care in the U.S. has never been distributed on the basis of principles of equality. Roughly 45 million non-elderly Americans were without health insurance in 2003.[50] Although this figure increased throughout the 1990s, lack of health insurance is a longstanding problem in this country. Many Americans are also underinsured. That is, they cannot, for example, afford the cost of drugs or the co-payment required to visit their general practitioner.[51] Moreover, many Americans seem to receive a compromised quality of care because they are black or poor.[52] There is also some evidence that African Americans have less trust in their physicians than do other Americans. They appear to be less satisfied with their 'experience' with their physicians' listening skills, explanations, and thoroughness.[53]

Managing care according to different health-plan specifications can erode the professional practice standard and further underscores differences in access to health-care resources, even among the insured. Neighbors living next to each other and colleagues within the same workplace will often have different health-care benefits. Some will have platinum plans while others have no-frills health care. Some patients will have to travel long distances to receive an MRI, while others visit their local hospital. Managed care as it is implemented in the U.S. exacerbates existing inequalities and may increase the perception of inequality by distributing care according to the plan in which one is enrolled. Thus, it highlights inequality with respect to health care.

Given the importance of peoples' bodies to their conceptions of 'self' and physical and emotional integrity, distributing health care unequally and according to what people will or can pay may create tension within the community. Inequalities in health care may weigh more heavily in how people view themselves and their place in the community than inequalities in the distribution of other goods. Margaret Somerville has the following to say:[54]

> Because we all personally relate to and identify with health care, it is a very important power for creating values, implementing those values and carrying them forward . . . thus health care is an ethics laboratory . . . . Our decisions about health care . . . have a much wider impact on society as a whole.

Managed care has underscored access issues by eroding the egalitarian impact of the professional practice standard. Under fee-for-service, health care was distributed to the insured based on need, as determined by a physician, informed by the professional practice standard.[55] Although some patients could pay for insurance that would buy them more prestigious physicians, in principle, all patients were entitled to care dictated by the professional practice standard.[56] In effect, the professional practice standard buttresses fiduciary ethics and an egalitarian approach to the distribution of health care, at least with respect to those who have health insurance. By influencing physicians' clinical behavior, managed care also influences the ability of physicians to treat patients on the basis of the standard of care. The ethical commitment to the principle that *all* patients should receive the same care given the same need, regardless of what they can afford, has been threatened by some reimbursement schemes.[57] Although the tendency of physicians to manipulate reimbursement rules to access benefits for their patients[58] may be viewed as evidence of their commitment to the idea that patients ought to receive the same care regardless of what health plan they have, it is also evidence of the difficulties they experience in implementing that commitment.

Under the current system, managed plans offer payers and subscribers different benefits at different costs. In this way, the decision about what treatment options are available to patients for particular conditions is decided prior to the onset of the relationship between doctor and patient. In Chapter 6, I explore the implications of this change for social capital. Managed health plans treat patients unequally insofar as they allocate care not solely on the basis of what patients need, as determined by their physicians in light of the professional practice standard. Instead, at their best, managed plans distribute health care to patients on the basis of what benefits are available under the plan patients are enrolled in.[59] Patients fortunate enough to have chosen more generous health plans would receive different and perhaps better treatment. Some people would argue that, under managed care, patients will be the recipients of a different kind of respect, one in which their wishes, as expressed in their choice of a health-care plan, are respected.[60]

Haavi Morreim seems to believe that patients in managed-care plans are respected thusly:[61]

> To hold a competent adult to the consequences of his own tradeoff decisions, even where this means informing him that he is not free to pursue certain [medical] options that he, himself, foreclosed . . . honors his autonomy by respecting the choices he made for his 'larger life'— not just the part of him that needs medical care.

Some of the adverse consequences of honoring these decisions will be felt most strongly by the poor, those who have already experienced the effects of disproportionate social status. They will find themselves in less generous health plans; they will not have available to them the benefits of being treated as a member of a privileged class, the money to walk away, secure a second opinion, or buy platinum class service. Moreover, the effects will be felt more deeply by them because they are already vulnerable and what is at issue, their health, carries great symbolic significance.[62] However, other harms associated with unequal social status will be shared by all.

Given the potential health value of equality, there are good reasons to reduce inequalities, especially in the important sphere of health care. Health plans that manage care have taken some resource allocation questions out of the hands of physicians and away from the relatively impartial test of the professional practice standard. Now decisions about patient care are determined by the various contingencies of shareholder demands, what employers are willing to pay, and what health plans have successfully negotiated. By tiering people's health care according to what benefits they can pay for, and by divorcing the distribution of health care from the professional practice standard, managed-health plans have violated the principle of universalism.

The myth of choice

Some bioethicists have tried to take the moral sting out of managed care by arguing that there is something morally suspect about providing people with more health care than they have paid for or indicated a desire for.[63] Haavi Morreim, for example, suggests that some subscribers may just want a basic, no-frills health plan and that, for example, they might prefer to spend their money on a ski trip.[64] No one would advocate that we force unwanted health care onto people. But providing people with the option to choose what care they need, free from financial worry, is not equivalent to insisting that they receive care against their wishes.

In any case, it is difficult to characterize the choice of health plans as 'free' when most subscribers receive their insurance at their workplace, many workplaces offer only one plan, and subscribers may not understand the terms of the plans.[65] But even if we assume, and I believe wrongly, that patients want 'no frills' health care, their preferences are not the only ones relevant. If, as I maintain, their choices adversely affect the community, then the community also has an interest in the health-care plans that individuals choose.

I have argued that some of the cost containment mechanisms employed by managed care, especially when implemented aggressively, undermine social relationships that are vital for health. Managing health care according to the benefits for which people pay also underscores differences in access to health care in an unprecedented way. Given the connection between health and equality, thusly managing health care has the potential to further compromise our health. In view of the research on social relations and equality, we need to be concerned that some managed care will exacerbate some of the social and health problems associated with inequality.

Notes

1 B. Weston and M. Lauria. Patient Advocacy in the 1990's. *New England Journal of Medicine*, 1996; 334: 543–4; B. Herbert. Torture by HMO. *New York Times*, 15 March 1996, §A, p. 29, col. 1.

2 Weston and Lauria, op. cit.; M. Guy. Policy Watch: Physicians and Patients Versus HMOs. *American Journal of Medicine*, 1996; 101: 1; Herbert, op. cit.

3 D.M. Fox. The Politics of Trust in American Health Care. In *Ethics, Trust, and The Professions*, ed. E. Pellegrino et al. Washington, DC: Georgetown University Press: 1991, pp. 3–22; W.K. Mariner. Business vs. Medical Ethics: Conflicting Standards for Managed Care. *Journal of Law, Medicine and Ethics*, 1995; 23: 241.

4 This would follow if the studies showing a connection between social support and health are right. L.F. Berkman. Social Networks and Health: The Bonds that Heal. In *The Society and Population Health Reader: A State and Community Perspective*, ed. A.R. Tarlov and R.F. St. Peter, Vol. 2, New York: New Press, 2000.

5 U.S.A. Today/CNN/Gallup Poll, 5–8 July 2002, as described in J.M. Jones. Poll Analyses: Americans Express Little Trust in CEOs of Large Corporations or Stockbrockers. *Gallup News Service*, 17 July 2002.

6 D.W. Brock. Broadening the Bioethics Agenda. *Kennedy Institute of Ethics Journal*, 2000; 10: 21–38.

7 For a good recent account of other interferences with medical trust see R. Rhodes. Trust and Transforming Medical Institutions. *Cambridge Quarterly of Healthcare Ethics*, 2000; 4: 205.

8 Berkman, op. cit., p. 260.

9 Ibid.

10 For a good overview of this material, see I. Kawachi. Social Cohesion and Health. In Tarlov and St Peter, op. cit., pp. 57–74.

11 S. Wolfe and J. Bruhn. *The Power of the Clan: A 25-year Prospective Study of Roseto, PA*, New Brunswick, NJ: Transaction Publishers, 1992; J. Bruhn and S. Wolfe. *The Roseto Story: An Anatomy of Health*. OK: Norman, University of Oklahoma Press, 1979.

12 Ibid.

13 E. Durkheim. *Suicide: A Study in Sociology*, ed. G. Simpson. tr. J.A. Spaulding and G. Simpson. New York: Free Press, 1951. As quoted in I. Kawachi and L. Berkman. Social Cohesion, Social Capital, and Health. In *Social Epidemiology*,

ed. I. Kawachi and L. Berkman. New York: Oxford University Press, 2000, p. 175.

14 Ibid.

15 Ibid.

16 U.S.A. Today/CNN/Gallup Poll, op. cit.

17 Berkman, op. cit., p. 260.

18 L.F. Berkman and S.L. Syme. Social Networks, Host Resistance and Mortality: a Nine Year Follow-up Study of Alameda County Residents. *American Journal of Epidemiology*, 1979; 109: 186–204.

19 Berkman, op. cit., p. 261.

20 D.G. Blazer. Social Support and Mortality in an Elderly Community Population. *American Journal of Epidemiology*, 1982; 115: 684–94.

21 S. Hoffman and M.C. Hatch. Stress, Social Support and Pregnancy Outcomes: A Reassessment Based on Recent Research. *Paediatric and Perinatal Epidemiology*, 1996; 10: 380–405.

22 W. Ruberman et al. Psychosocial Influences on Mortality After Myocardial Infarction. *New England Journal of Medicine*, 1984; 311: 552–9.

23 K. Ortho-Gomer et al. Social Isolation and Mortality in Ischemic Heart Disease. *Acta Medical School*, 1988; 224: pp. 205–15; see also R.B. Williams et al. Prognostic: Importance of Social and Economic Resources Among Medically Treated Patients with Angiographically Documented Coronary Heart Disease. *Journal of the American Medical Association*, 1992; 267: 520–4; R.B. Case et al. Living Alone After Myocardial Infarction. *Journal of the American Medical Association*, 1992; 267: 515. For a good critical review of the literature on the social determinants of health, see T.E. Seeman. Social Ties and Health: The Benefits of Social Integration. *Annals of Epidemiology*, 1996; 6: 442–51.

24 Berkman, op. cit., p. 265.

25 L.F. Berkman. The Changing and Heterogeneous Nature of Aging and Longevity. *Annual Review of Gerontology and Geriatrics*, 1988; 8: 37–68.

26 D.W. Brock. Broadening the Bioethics Agenda. *Kennedy Institute of Ethics Journal*, 2000; 10: 22.

27 Berkman, op. cit., p. 272.

28 Ibid., p. 273.

29 See, for example, the commentary by W.T. Branch. Is the Therapeutic Nature of the Patient–Physician Relationship Being Undermined? A Primary Care Physician's Perspective. *Archives of Internal Medicine*, 2000; 160: 2257–60.

30 American Nursing Association. Nursing's Social Policy Statement. Washington, DC: American Nurses Publishing, 1995. In Joanne Reitter-Teital. The Impact of Restructuring Professional Nursing Administration. *Journal of Nursing Administration* 2002; 32: 31–41.

31 K. Grumbach et al. Resolving the Gatekeeper Conundrum: What Patients Value in Primary Care and Referrals to Specialists. *Journal of the American Medical Association*, 1999; 282: 264; E.A. Kern et al. The Influence of Gatekeeping and Utilization Review on Patient Satisfaction. *Journal of General Internal Medicine*, 1999; 14: 287–96.

32 Kaiser Family Foundation. *Kaiser Public Opinion Update*, August 2001, showing that the majority of those surveyed believe that managed care has decreased access to specialists, time with doctors, and the quality of care for the sick, Grumbach et al., op. cit., pp. 261–6.

33 The rise of luxury practices may signal an effort to recapture some of these. T. Brennan. Luxury Primary Care—Market Innovation or Threat to Access? *New England Journal of Medicine*, 2002; 346: 1165–8.

34 S. Dorr Goold. Money and Trust: Relationships between Patients, Physicians, and Health Plans. *Journal of Health Politics, Policy and Law*, 1998; 23: 687–95.

35 A. Wu et al. Quality of Care and Outcomes of Adults with Asthma Treated by Specialists and Generalists in Managed Care. *Archives of Internal Medicine*, 2001; 161: 2554–60.

36 T.E. Miller and W. Sage. Disclosing Physician Financial Incentives. *Journal of the American Medical Association*, 1999; 281: 1425.

37 See L.J. Weiss and J. Blustein. Faithful Patients: The Effect of Long-Term Physician–Patient Relationships on the Costs and Use of Health Care by Older Americans. *American Journal of Public Health*, 1996; 86: 1742–7; M.M. Love et al. Continuity of Care and the Physician–Patient Relationship. *Journal of Family Practice*, 2000; 49: 998–1004.

38 D. Mechanic. Models of Rationing: Professional Judgment and the Rationing of Medical Care, 140 *University of Pennsylvania Law Review* 1713, May 1992.

39 Interestingly, it also appears that 'social relatedness' makes people happy and satisfies a strong psychological need. If so, and there is evidence to support this, a doctor–patient relationship that fosters connectedness has the potential to not only make patients healthy, but happy. From a consequentialist perspective, this is an important advantage of a trust-rich doctor–patient relationship. See: K.M. Sheldon et al., What is Satisfying about Satisfying Events? Testing Ten Candidate Psychological Needs. *Journal of Personality and Social Psychology*, 2001; 80: 329.

40 F. Diderichsen et al. The Social Basis of Disparities in Health. In *Social Epidemiology*, ed. I. Kawachi and L. Berkman. Oxford: Oxford University Press, 2000, pp. 13–23; E. Backlund et al. The Shape of the Relationship Between Income and Mortality in the United States: Evidence from the National Longitudinal Mortality Study. *Annals of Epidemiology*, 1996; 6: 12–20.

41 R.G. Wilkinson. Social Relations, Hierarchy, and Health. In *The Society and Population Health Reader: A State and Community Perspective*, Vol. 2, ed. I. Kawachi et al. New York: The New Press, 1999, pp. 211–35.

42 For a good discussion of the ethical implications, see N. Daniels et al. Justice, Health and Health Policy. In *Ethical Dimensions of Health Policy*, ed. M. Davis et al. New York: Oxford University Press, 2002, pp. 19–47.

43 For a good overview, see I. Kawachi et al. Introduction. In *The Society and Population Health Reader: Income Inequality and Health*, Vol. 1, ed. I. Kawachi et al. New York: The New Press, 1999, pp. xi–xxxvi.

44 See G.B. Rogers. Income and Inequality as Determinants of Mortality: An International Cross-Section Analysis. in *The Society and Population Health Reader: Income Inequality and Health*, Vol. 1, op. cit., pp. 5–13; R.J. Waldmann. Income Distribution and Infant Mortality. In *The Society and Population Health Reader: Income Inequality and Health*, Vol. 1, op. cit., pp. 14–27; R.G. Wilkinson. Income Distribution and Life Expectancy. In *The Society and Population Health Reader: Income Inequality and Health*, Vol. 1, op. cit., pp. 28–35.

45 R.G. Wilkinson. Health, Hierarchy, and Social Anxiety. *Annals of the New York Academy of Sciences*, 1999; 896: 48–63.

46 C.A. Shively et al. The Behavior and Physiology of Social Stress and Depression in Female Cynomolgus Monkeys. *Biological Psychiatry*, 1997; 41: 871–2.

47 The Whitehall II study was a 1985–88 follow-up to the 1967 original Whitehall study, which measured mortality of British civil servants according to their grade of employment. Whitehall II showed a steep inverse relationship between

social class/employment rank and health status. In addition, Marmot et al. found an inverse association, according to employment rank, with employees' health, economic situation, and satisfaction with work (as characterized by degree of control at work). See M.G. Marmot et al. Health Inequalities Among British Civil Servants: the Whitehall II Study. *The Lancet,* 1991; 337: 1387–93.

48 M.G. Marmot et al. Contributions of Job Control and Other Social Variations in Coronary Heart Disease Incidence. *The Lancet,* 1997; 350: 235–9.

49 K.M. Sheldon et al. What's Satisfying About Satisfying Events? Testing Ten Candidate Psychological Needs. *Journal of Personality and Social Psychology,* 2001; 80: 329.

50 C. DeNavas-Walt et al. Income, Poverty, and Health Insurance Coverage in the United States: 2003. *Current Population Reports* of U.S. Census Bureau Department of Commerce Economics, and Statistics Administration, August 2004, p.14.

51 Kaiser Family Foundation. Kaiser Commission on Medicaid and the Uninsured Key Facts on Underinsured in America: Is Health Coverage Adequate? July 2002.

52 See, for example, E.D. Peterson et al. Racial Variation in the Use of Coronary Revascularization Procedures: Are the Differences Real? Do They Matter? *New England Journal of Medicine,* 1997; 336: 480–6; J.M. Mitchell et al. Access to Bone Marrow Transplantation for Leukemia and Lymphoma: The Role of Sociodemographic Factors. *Journal of Clinical Oncology,* 1997; 15: 2644–51. See also C. Kahn et al. Health Care for Black and Poor Hospitalized Medicare Patients. *Journal of the American Medical Association,* 1994; 271: 1169–74.

53 M.P. Doescher et al. Racial and Ethnic Disparities in Perceptions of Physician Style and Trust. *Archives of Family Medicine,* 2000; 9: 1156–63.

54 M. Somerville. *The Ethical Canary.* Toronto: Viking Press, 2000, p. 4.

55 Some might argue that the professional practice standard does not directly inform physicians' medical decisions—but it is a standard of legal liability. Arguably, however, it does both; physicians are liable under it and practice in the shadow of it.

56 Although this may strike some people as an insignificant right given the number of uninsured, another way to view it is as a first step in the direction of substantive care for all.

57 The professional practice standard is the tort standard to which physicians are subject to suit for medical malpractice. According to this standard, physicians have a duty to deliver the same care that other physicians in the same community deliver. Note that the standard is not conditional upon the patients having the same resources available. If we transpose this from a duty to an entitlement, then it would be fair to say that patients are entitled to receive the same care as other patients. Managed care has disrupted this by participating in medical decisions and deciding what to cover according to what people pay. For an excellent discussion, see E.H. Morreim. *Holding Health Care Accountable.* New York: Oxford University Press, 2001.

58 M.K. Wynia et al. Physician Manipulation of Reimbursement Rules for Patients: Between a Rock and a Hard Place. *Journal of the American Medical Association,* 2000; 238: 1858–65.

59 Determining what patients actually receive in managed plans is complex since what is received may depend on a variety of factors, including in a capitated system the capitated amount. For the discussion of availability of resources, see the definition of managed care in Chapter 1.

60 E.H. Morreim. *Balancing Act: The New Medical Ethics of Medicine's New Economics.* Washington, DC: Georgetown University Press, 1995; A.A. Stone. Paradigms, Pre-emptions, and Stages: Understanding the Transformation of

American Psychiatry by Managed Care. *International Journal of Law and Psychiatry*, 1995; 18: 353–87; W.K. Mariner. Business vs. Medical Ethics: Conflicting Standards for Managed Care. *Journal of Law, Medicine and Ethics*, 1995; 23: 240.

61 Morreim, op. cit., p. 142.
62 Kawachi et al., op. cit., p. xxxi.
63 Morreim, op. cit., p. 143; courts have used consent to justify some of the cost containment mechanisms used by managed care. See, for example, *Shea v. Eisenstein* 208 F.3d 712 (8th Cir 2000) and *Ward v. Alternative Health Delivery System* 55 F. Supp. 2d 694, 699 (2000).
64 Morreim, op. cit., p. 142.
65 M.A. Hall et al. How Disclosing HMO Physician Incentives Affects Trust. *Health Affairs*, 2002; 21: 197; Kaiser Family Foundation. *Chartbook: Trends and Indicators in the Changing Health Care Marketplace*, May 2002, Exhibit 2.4.

5 Conserving medical trust for the sake of social capital

Our health is affected by the quality of community life.[1] This consists of a web of social relationships, including the relationship patients have with their physicians and other providers. As already noted, there is good evidence that the more extensive our social network, the better our health. Similarly, studies indicate that above a certain level of income, the more equality these relations reflect, the healthier we will be. The doctor–patient relationship is important as a source of medical care and, as I have argued, an important social relationship nestled in a web of relationships.[2] Thus, in addition to providing needed health care, the doctor–patient relationship has the wherewithal to contribute to the richness of community life. The benefits of the relationship between doctor and patient are not conferred solely on patients, but extend widely to the community in the form of social capital.[3]

The concept of 'social capital' has a long and distinguished history, beginning in the early twentieth century when it was used by education reformers to encourage participation in schools.[4] According to J. Coleman,[5]

> social capital is defined by its function. It is not a single entity, but a variety of different entities claiming two characteristics in common: they all consist of some aspect of social structure, and they facilitate certain actions of individuals who are within the structure. Like other forms of capital, social capital is productive, making possible the achievement of certain ends that would not be attainable in its absence.

More recently, the concept of 'social capital' has been popularized by Francis Fukayama and Robert Putnam.[6] It is also widely used in public health analyses by social epidemiologists. Ichiro Kawachi and Lisa Berkman have noted two generalizations common to various definitions of 'social capital.' First, that social capital is social. That is, it is 'a feature of the collective (neighborhood, community, society) to which the individual belongs.'[7] Second, it is a public good. Moreover, it should be viewed as a 'byproduct of social relationships.'[8]

The concept of 'social capital' can also be understood by looking at what it produces. Social capital creates the possibility of productive, cooperative activity. According to Putnam, social capital consists in 'the networks, norms, and social trust that facilitate coordination and cooperation for mutual benefit.'[9] For Putnam, important indicators of social capital are levels of trust, perceived reciprocity, and the extent of membership in civic associations. Social capital can be viewed as one of the benefits 'that flow from the trust, reciprocity, information, and cooperation associated with social networks. Social capital creates value for the people who are connected and at least sometimes for bystanders.'[10] Although a number of people have written about social capital, I will, for the most part, rely on Putnam's account. The application of his theoretical work to the American context coincides with some of my analysis on health care in the U.S.

Three important indicators of social capital are: (1) norms, values, and attitudes, (2) networks, and (3) consequences.[11] Trust is a crucial attitude for the creation of social capital. It has the potential to transform self-interested and self-seeking actors into collaborators and cooperators. Because of this, the extent of trust in a relationship is often a good measure of the degree of social capital present. Trust facilitates generalized reciprocity. In turn, generalized reciprocity takes interpersonal relations outside of a tit-for-tat exchange in which people require an immediate return on their 'gifts.' When people are part of a community in which generalized reciprocity is abundant, they know that they will be a beneficiary at some later time and perhaps from another person. It isn't necessary for them to exact reciprocation for their gift at the time it is given. Without trust, generalized reciprocity would be impossible and without generalized reciprocity, there would be little or no social capital. The willingness of people to undertake a burden, such as watering their neighbors' plants while they are on vacation, hinges on trusting that they or someone else will extend the same or a similar kindness in the future.

Networks can be a very tangible form of social capital, as in the case of an extensive list of personal and professional contacts. People with wide networks more effectively advance themselves professionally and socially. And as we know from our analysis of social relations, social networks are important for individual health and well-being. Because networks convey the message that strangers can be 'relied on' for kindness, they also create social capital for the community.[12] Social capital is thought to have a number of positive consequences, including 'mutual support, cooperation, trust and institutional effectiveness.'[13] It has been found to be important for preventing delinquency, improving education and community life, and in criminology.[14]

Two different kinds of social capital have been identified, 'bonding' and 'bridging.' Bonding social capital reinforces the inward perspective of a group, and it can be found in homogenous groups, such as fraternal organizations.[15] Unlike bridging social capital, social capital of this kind can breed exclusivity among relatively insular groups. Nonetheless, it provides support for members of the group. It is facilitated by the 'thick trust' of face-to-face interactions within primary relations.[16]

Bridging social capital, facilitated by thin trust, is the glue that links people among different groups to each other. Thin trust, unlike thick trust, fosters a willingness to trust people outside of our immediate circle.[17] Bridging social capital is valuable precisely because it builds bridges between groups and enhances the willingness of people 'to give most people—even those whom they do not know from direct experience—the benefit of the doubt.'[18] Because bridging social capital promotes tolerance and empathy it is particularly important in a society as diverse as ours.

Trust and social capital

Trust and social capital go hand in hand. According to Fukuyama, social capital is 'a capability that arises from the prevalence of trust in a society.'[19] It is facilitated by the shared norms permitting 'regular and honest cooperative behavior.'[20] Fukuyama cites the doctor–patient relationship as an example of the interplay between trust and values. He writes, '[We] trust a doctor not to do us deliberate injury because we expect him or her to live by the Hippocratic Oath and standards of the medical profession.'[21] Moreover, trust facilitates generalized reciprocity, which is the touchstone of social capital. Social capital should be understood as the product of cooperation among people, and cooperation depends on the existence of trust. Trust is therefore an important indicator of social capital.

Trust is also a social good. According to Sisella Bok, '[t]rust is a social good to be protected just as much as the air we breathe or the water we drink. When it is damaged, the community as a whole suffers and when it is destroyed, societies falter and collapse.'[22] A similar theme appears in much of the literature on social capital. Social capital and trust are non-excludable. They are genuine public goods insofar as social relations create them indirectly, and the benefits from them cannot be restricted to those who, themselves, have contributed to their cultivation. Free riders, individuals, and institutions, who for example have not contributed to the 'trust fund,' can nonetheless draw on its wealth. The relationship between trust and social capital is complex. Trust is a component or mark of social capital, but is also independent of it.

Let us try to place the doctor–patient relationship within the framework of thick and thin trust. Although it would seem most naturally to fall within the category of thin trust, because of the potential for infrequent visits to the physician, the trust of the doctor–patient relationship is an interesting hybrid. Thick trust is typically associated with relationships that involve regular, frequent interactions, such as those one might have with the postman. Thick trust is founded in our unique experience with a particular person. Thin trust is prized because it facilitates interactions among people who don't know each other. Patients appear to be able to trust their physicians without frequent personal interaction, perhaps in part because of the values the physician places on universal care.[23] Yet what could be more personal than discussing the various illnesses that plague one's body?

The doctor–patient relationship seems to be a source of both thick trust and, more importantly, thin trust. It creates bonds, and it builds bridges. In this respect, it outshines many other significant sources of trust. The trust that evolves within the doctor–patient relationship is especially valuable because it suggests that even people we meet only infrequently can be trusted with what many people value deeply—their health and the health of their loved ones.

Thin trust is also a scarcer resource than thick trust. The fact that thick trust is based on frequent interactions, as in families and partnerships, means that there will be other opportunities to either exact the sought after 'good' or to seek punishment and revenge when trust is breached. In some sense, trust is less important in these contexts than it is when social relations are infrequent. Trust is also crucial for large organizations.[24]

Social capital is prized because of the benefits it produces for both individuals and communities. Studies have shown that people with high levels of trust volunteer more often, contribute more to charity, participate in civic and community organizations, serve on juries, and comply with tax obligations.[25] Trust and social capital also have health benefits. According to researchers 'lower levels of social trust were associated with most major causes of death'.[26] Also, individuals living in states with low social capital are more likely to rate themselves as having poor health.[27] Kawachi attributes the connection between low social capital and poor health outcomes to three possible causes: (1) social capital influences health-related behaviors, (2) social capital influences access to services and amenities, and (3) social capital affects psychosocial processes.[28] Even if social capital is responsible for only a portion of these social goods, it would be a commodity worth protecting.

Engagement and connectedness, two characteristics of social capital, are present in the doctor–patient relationship.[29] Although professional distance is an important trait for physicians, physicians can experience and express deep concern for the welfare of their patients. Together, physicians and patients may share the joy of birth, the grief associated with loss, and the fear of death. In this way, they can make connections with each other that are deep and lasting. It would not be surprising if connectedness and engagement are at least part of what makes continuity of care so important to patients.[30] For some people, including the elderly, the relationships with their physicians are important and may be among the relatively few relationships they have that are trust based (among the elderly other social ties often disappear).[31]

The consequences of diminishing social capital for individuals

If my analysis is right and trust confers benefits on those who have it, then patients in lower-trust doctor–patient relationships are likely to be worse off than those in high-trust relationships. Many patients may require high levels of trust in their physicians in order to make the kinds of disclosures that are required for accurate and timely diagnosis and to comply with 'doctor's orders.'[32] According to one study, 85 percent of the information physicians use for patient diagnosis is derived from patients.[33] Whether or not patients provide physicians with the information they need may depend on the quality of the relationship.[34] Many patients may lose the therapeutic benefits of a high-trust relationship.[35]

Furthermore, given the importance of trust in general, patients who have lower levels of trust because of their experience in the doctor–patient relationship may be disadvantaged in other areas of their lives. If trust, as others and I have argued, also has important social dimensions, and the doctor–patient relationship is a significant source of trust, then diminishing this stock of trust will reverberate in the community. In Chapters 2 and 3, I argued that some managed care, cost containment mechanisms have the potential to put trust between doctor and patient at risk. Given a conceptual understanding of social capital, lower trust in both doctors and the health-care system may have an adverse impact on social capital. This follows to some extent from a conceptual analysis of both trust and social capital. Since the degree of social capital present in a community is related to the degree of trust present, including trust between doctor and patient, less of one will affect the other and vice versa. More concretely, lower levels of trust among individuals may, for example, make one reluctant to engage in the 'dance' of generalized reciprocity and this, in turn, may adversely impact social capital.

There has been little empirical research on the connection between provider trust and social capital. A very recent study, however, finds a positive association between social capital and physician trust. In this study, Ahern and Hendryx found that increased general trust in the community (a component of social capital) was positively associated with trust in providers.[36] More specifically, trust in HMO physicians was less negatively affected when patients lived in communities rich in social capital. Given this association between social capital and trust, and the theoretical connection between trust and social capital, it is likely that a reciprocal relationship exists. That is, just as higher levels of social capital in our community affect trust in the doctor–patient relationship, so lower levels of trust in the doctor–patient relationship may adversely affect levels of social capital. In other words, the relationship between 'medical trust' and social capital is a cyclical one.[37] In the face of aggressively managed plans and a decline in medical trust, the relationship between doctor and patient threatens to erode social capital. The loss of trust from this source is important, not only because of the consequences that follow when it is withdrawn, but also because of the relative scarcity of trust in the community.[38] Trust and social capital are difficult to come by, and we can ill afford to lose them.

Harm to the community from our depleted fund of social capital

There are few relationships today in which people invest as much trust as patients traditionally have in their doctors.[39] And although it may be disadvantageous for patients to trust physicians who are undeserving of their trust, trust in trustworthy physicians has direct benefits for patients as well as indirect benefits for the community.[40] Trust generates trust.[41] An implication of the economic account of 'trust' is that the more instances of successful trusting that people have, the more they will be able to trust others both in and out of the medical context. Trust can be converted into social capital, which, in turn, facilitates successful cooperative and mutually beneficial activity within the community. In this way, it is self-reinforcing and enhances both interpersonal relationships and community life.

Because the doctor–patient relationship is a unique hybrid of thick and thin trust and bonding social capital, it is worth speculating that losing trust here may carry with it a greater loss than other instances of depleted trust. Instead of reassuring patients that strangers can be relied on for kindness, a hallmark of bridging social capital, physicians practicing in aggressive managed care may confirm their patients' worst fears that they will not, for example, be cared for, be referred to needed specialists, or have their interests be primary.[42]

To identify the harms that would be borne by the community because of this loss of trust, we need only reflect on the benefits to be had from social capital. First and most important are the benefits associated with cooperative activity. Without social capital, problems that require a collective solution will either remain unresolved or require elaborate and more expensive legal mechanisms.[43] But we may lose more than efficient problem solving. Opportunities for new ideas and the creative projects that arise out of co-operative activity may also be lost. Second, high levels of trust can have economic benefits for businesses and the community.[44] Thus reduced trust from the doctor–patient relationship may be reflected in economic externalities.[45] Third, diminished social capital may compromise the characteristics that make people socially valuable members of the community. They may be less tolerant and less empathic of others.[46] The community also stands to lose with respect to children's welfare and the health of all.[47] Thus, the harmful consequences of diminished trust within the doctor–patient relationship will be felt beyond the health concerns of individual patients.

Ironically, managed-health plans themselves may find that they endure a unique burden because of reduced social capital. Ahern and Hendryx speculate that improved social capital in the community may facilitate trust between providers and patients associated with HMOs. Such trust will of course reduce the greater transaction costs associated with distrust for health plans.[48]

In the event of a depletion of trust, it is likely that certain segments of the community will be injured more deeply than others because they already experience lower levels of trust. In addition, these segments do not have access to the finances to compensate for their deprivation.[49] The poor, for example, may have diminished access to social capital and may have lower levels of trust than the wealthy.[50] People who have had a high number of trust-eroding experiences, such as the victims of childhood abuse, will be at greater risk than those who have had a relatively strong, trust-building childhood. Moreover, the wealthy are in a position to purchase trust-building experiences, perhaps by way of pricey psychotherapy, or through the services of a lawyer who can ensure reciprocity.[51]

It is also worth keeping in mind that social capital appears to be a relatively scarce resource. Social disengagement is widespread. Participation in the various organizations that foster social capital has steadily declined over the last few decades. Robert Putnam has documented this decline, showing reduced levels of civic participation and social engagement over the last 30 years. Civic and social participation in the affairs of the community helps to create social capital by increasing the frequency of interaction among people and thus contributing to the likelihood of generalized reciprocity.[52] Thus, reduced participation may precipitate reduced social capital. According to Putnam, the number of people agreeing that most people can be trusted fell from 58 percent in 1960 to 37 percent in 1993.[53]

The argument that the doctor–patient relationship is an important source of trust and social capital does not depend on showing that trust and social capital are declining. Nonetheless, knowing that our general reservoir of social capital is diminishing should serve to increase our appreciation of available sources and caution us against squandering what remains.[54] Granted the doctor–patient relationship is not the only source of trust and social capital. There are many others. All of us interact daily with a number of people from different lifestyles, and some people may rarely see their physicians. Although trust can be found in a number of relationships, and social capital can accumulate incrementally from many of them, the doctor–patient relationship is among a relatively few 'high-trust' relationships.[55]

Unlike a relationship with, for example, the grocer, the doctor–patient relationship requires high levels of trust to be successful.[56] There is more trust to lose in the doctor–patient relationship, and its loss can have a greater impact. Grocers may be more easily replaced than physicians. Medical care may also have a symbolic significance, such that it generates social capital, even at a distance. People may not need to visit their physicians for the relationship to generate trust. Finally, although social capital accumulates from a variety of sources, and each source contributes to the reservoir, some sources will make greater contributions than others. In all likelihood, the doctor–patient relationship makes a greater contribution to our fund of social capital than does, for example, the grocer–client relationship.

Although the aftermath of the tragedy of 11 September 2001 brought with it an upswing in both trust and social capital, we should not be lulled into false optimism. According to Putnam, much of the post 9/11 civic engagement is expressed in rhetoric and images and not in ongoing civic participation.[57] Thus far it has not resulted in policies that would foster inclusion and cultivate trust and social capital.

Implications for the consent argument

It is possible to consistently acknowledge the weaknesses with aggressively implemented managed care and at the same time defend it on moral grounds. Arguably, subscribers to health plans have consented to the quality and kind of care that they receive.[58] According to this line of reasoning when people subscribe to a health plan they consent not only to the specific benefits in the plan, but also to the level of trust that the plan permits.[59] The persuasiveness of this argument hinges on a fiction. First, many people are offered only one health plan.[60] Second, chances are that few people are even aware of the harm that can befall them from erosion of trust and social capital. Third, and most importantly, even if (1) they are aware of the potential for harm to themselves and to the community, and (2) they are entitled on the basis of autonomy considerations to 'harm' themselves, they are not entitled to consent to harms to the community.[61] It is not theirs to consent to. Although individuals can consent to 'harm' to themselves, they do not have the right to consent to harm to others unless it has been explicitly given to them either through consent or a special relationship.[62] In Mill's words, '[a]s soon as any part of a person's conduct affects prejudicially the interests of others, society has jurisdiction over it, and the question whether the general welfare will or will not be promoted by interfering with it, becomes open to discussion.'[63]

A consideration of trust and social capital shows that the community has an investment in the relationships and institutions that produce trust and facilitate social capital. If medical trust is a public good, then individuals do not have the moral right to trade health care rich in medical trust for trust-impoverished health care any more than they have the moral right to purchase a low-cost car that spews high levels of toxic fumes. Just as we recognize a need to intervene in organizational behavior in order to protect natural resources such as clean air and water, so too do we have an interest and a duty to protect our social resources, such as social capital. The doctor–patient relationship is in this respect a public good. But a note of caution is in order. I am not advocating that the community always has a right to intervene in conduct that adversely affects social capital. In the case at hand, however, it is difficult to view the interest in maintaining a low-trust doctor–patient relationship as compelling. The decision about what activities to intervene in on behalf of social capital and what activities to tolerate despite their cost to social capital will require a balancing of interests. In the case of medical trust, the interest that some may believe that they have in a low-trust relationship may be overshadowed by the need to pool risks with others, the nature of medicine as a social institution, and the questionable value of the interest in a low-trust doctor–patient relationship.[64]

Protecting our reservoir of medical trust

We are now well positioned to consider the moral arguments in support of maintaining a doctor–patient relationship that fosters trust and social capital. Whenever conduct harms others, the community may incur a duty to regulate that conduct. This follows from John Stuart Mill's famous harm principle.[65] Roughly, that principle states that one ought never to interfere with a person's self-regarding actions, but only with the actions that harm other people.[66] One of the grounds for objecting to health plans that impair trust between doctor and patient, such as aggressively implemented capitation, is that they also interfere with the community's trust fund. When an action or activity causes harm to others, the usual autonomy-based prohibition against interfering with it is lifted. The idea behind this is that the liberty of some should not be purchased at the cost of the liberty of others. A moral duty to conserve a high-trust relationship between doctor and patient can be justified given the moral imperative to protect the community from harm to its fund of social capital. But there are other moral arguments that speak for a high-trust doctor–patient relationship.

First, consider the moral minimum, do no harm.[67] The principle of beneficence asks us at the least not to cause harm to others' valued goods. According to William Frankena, there are four dimensions to the principle: (1) a principle of nonmaleficence—one ought not to inflict harm, (2) one ought to prevent harm, (3) one ought to remove harm, and (4) one ought to promote good.[68] When aggressively managed care erodes the medical trust fund, it not only harms socially important goods, such as trust and social capital, it also increases the likelihood of poorer health outcomes.[69] Some health-care plans increase the likelihood of harm and in so doing violate the principle of beneficence.

Second, insofar as health plans erode the trust fund, they violate their consequentialist duties to produce good outcomes.[70] Trust and social capital cultivation are important mechanisms for producing good outcomes. Thus, aggressively managed care may harm the community by undermining an important source of trust and the potential to contribute to our reservoir of social capital. Managed care, at least when practiced aggressively, does little to improve our funds of trust and social capital—both of which foster good consequences. It may send utility spiraling downward.

Third, health plans that erode trust are free riders. At the same time that they enjoy the benefits of social capital, they deplete it. Some health plans draw on the wealth of social capital currently in the doctor–patient relationship by either explicitly or implicitly characterizing themselves as patient-centered as opposed to profit driven, and by piggybacking on the high esteem with which patients regard physicians.[71] Moreover, Ahern and Hendryx found an association between increased social capital and increased provider trust.[72] Insofar as trust between doctor and patient facilitates the care of patients, it would seem to be in the interest of health plans to have more rather than less of it. Health plans that draw on our fund of social capital without contributing to it violate principles of fair play. But more importantly, this behavior shows that some plans are not entitled to the share of social capital that they have taken. When it comes to social capital some health plans may be 'in the red' and, arguably, owe the community compensation for the social capital they have taken without reciprocation. To use Putnam's words, they have not participated in generalized reciprocity. Finally, insofar as health plans erode social capital levels and do not contribute in turn, they have wrongly taken what does not belong to them, and in the case of for-profit plans, they have done so on behalf of shareholders. Social capital from the doctor–patient relationship is an important resource for the community and for future generations.

However, it is not just that aggressively managed plans have drawn on our fund of social capital without reciprocating in kind. They are not mere 'free riders.' If I am right, then aggressively practiced managed care has the potential to deplete the available trust from the doctor–patient relationship, making it difficult for others to access it at all. In other words, if aggressively managed medicine continues on the same trajectory, patients may find it increasingly difficult to trust their physicians.

An important liberty-based counter argument to the position I have developed in this book is that by regulating the doctor–patient relationship in the name of trust and social capital, we put another more important value at risk, individual liberty. Presumably, the liberty at issue here is the liberty to contract the services of a physician who is less expensive and less trustworthy. But surely this is shortsighted. Patients/subscribers often secure their health insurance through their employers, who often offer only one plan.[73] Given this, subscribers are not necessarily exercising liberty when they enroll in a plan. For regulation to involve a deprivation of liberty there must have been liberty in the first place. Today the choice of a health plan rarely entails much liberty. Moreover, by protecting trust within the doctor–patient relationship, liberty will be enhanced because people will have the wherewithal to take advantage of the full array of opportunities that become available because of the fund of social capital. Thus increased trust enhances positive liberty insofar as it enables people to achieve their ends.[74]

Trading trust

A number of scholars, including Allen Buchanan, have argued in support of replacing the bygone days of trust between doctor and patient with trust in health-care organizations. One important question to ask, assuming that such an exchange were possible, is whether trust in health-care organizations has the same potential to produce social capital, or indeed, to produce something preferable to social capital.

Although social capital may be important for determining the success of social institutions, institutions are not a particularly efficient mechanism for producing social capital.[75] According to some sociological literature, it is not easy to create social capital, especially within organizations. Large, formal, and especially hierarchical organizations are not useful in creating social capital in part because they do not occasion opportunities for interaction among members.[76] According to Putnam, social capital develops through 'habits of the heart' that arise in horizontal associations and informal groups, such as support groups and book clubs.[77]

Health-care organizations do not fall into this category. They are large hierarchical organizations in which face-to-face interactions are rare. Instead of a face-to-face dialog with a physician with whom one has a long-standing relationship, patients may well see a video or receive a pamphlet describing their condition. Members are more likely to encounter automated and recorded voices over the phone than the reassuring voice of a doctor or nurse. Moreover, health-care organizations are not horizontal organizations, but vertical ones, in which hierarchy prevails. When care is denied, patients will need to start down the long road to appeal. In any case, although this may be a fruitful way of ensuring procedural fairness, it is not promising with respect to social capital. Thus, as a society we find ourselves in the position where today's health plans are transforming the doctor–patient relationship from one that produced trust and social capital to one that may be incapable of doing so.

Some people would argue that managed care is serving an important social purpose by reducing unnecessary clinical spending and, in turn, increasing access to health care.[78] It is difficult to view the maximizing of corporate profits as stemming the costs of health care since often MCOs simply shift the cost of care to someone else. In the case at hand, there is an additional cost, namely, fidelity to patients and the benefits that this professionalism brings to the community. But the main problem with the access-to-care argument is that it just seems to be wrong. As it turned out, managed care actually did not in the end curb escalating health-care costs. Premiums for employer health insurance rose slightly in the mid-1990s, with a low of 9.8 percent in 1996 to 11.0 percent in 2001. Moreover, workers' earnings have increased only very slightly.[79] There is evidence that declines in health-care spending have been temporary and are followed by a rapid growth in costs.[80]

In the current health-care system, individual MCOs need not worry about the long-term consequences of their cost containment efforts since they may not deliver care to the same patients in the future. This point highlights a problem with managed care as it now stands. On the one hand, MCOs may be motivated by short-term gain, yet many health problems take years to materialize and become chronic conditions. Indeed, in capitated systems there is a risk that patients with chronic conditions will be deselected.[81]

There may not be adequate financial incentives for organizations primarily motivated by short-term economic gain to adequately address the many diseases that take years to present themselves. This holds for many of the diseases associated with differentiated social status. The effects of chronic stress on the human body, or differential social status, take time.[82] Moreover, since payers are usually employers, and employees frequently change jobs, employers have little incentive to pay the higher costs of the medical care needed to treat chronic conditions and that may ultimately benefit other employers or retired employees.[83] Social capital is an important social good, and the doctor–patient relationship has been a valuable vessel of trust, the main ingredient in social capital. Whether or not we will have to be satisfied with something less than a trust-rich doctor–patient relationship is still to be seen. We should not, however, be deceived into believing that we can simply trade our trust in physicians for trust in organizations and maintain the same benefits. We cannot.

Notes

1 L. Berkman. Social Networks and Health: The Bonds that Heal. In *The Society and Population Health Reader: A State and Community Perspective*, Vol. 2, ed. A.R. Tarlow and R.F. St Peter. New York: The Free Press, 2000, pp. 257–72; D.G. Blazer. Social Support and Mortality in an Elderly Community Population. *American Journal of Epidemiology*, 1982; 115: 684–94.
2 J.T. Hart and P. Dieppe. Caring Effects. *The Lancet*, 1996; 347: 1606–8.
3 For a similar perspective as applied not to physicians but to health systems, see L. Gilson. Trust and the Development of Health Care as a Social Institution. *Social Science and Medicine*, 2003; 56: 1453–68; for a critical review of the concept of social capital, see J. Macinko and B. Starfield. The Utility of Social Capital in Research on Health Determinants. *Milbank Quarterly*, 2001; 79: 387–427.
4 R. Putnam. *Bowling Alone*. New York: Simon & Schuster, 2000, p. 19.
5 J.S. Coleman. Social Capital in the Creation of Human Capital. *American Journal of Sociology*, 1988; 94 (Suppl.): 302.
6 F. Fukuyama. *Trust: The Social Virtues and The Creation of Prosperity*. New York: The Free Press, 1995; Putnam, op. cit.
7 I. Kawachi and L. Berkman. Social Cohesion, Social Capital, and Health. In *Social Epidemiology*, ed. L. Berkman and I. Kawachi. New York: Oxford University Press, 2000, pp. 176–7.
8 Ibid.
9 Putnam, op. cit., pp. 20–1.

10 The Saguaro Seminar: Civic Engagement in America. Social Capital Research: What is Social Capital? Online, available at: <http://www.ksg.harvard.edu/saguaro/primer.htm> (accessed 15 September 2004).

11 K. Newton. Social Capital and Democracy. *American Behavioral Scientist*, 1997; 40: 575.

12 Putnam, op. cit., p. 20.

13 Ibid., p. 22.

14 See M. Woolcock. Social Capital and Economic Development: Toward a Theoretical Synthesis and Policy Framework. *Theory and Society*, 1998; 27: 151–208; see also Kawachi and Berkman, op. cit., p. 174.

15 Putnam, op. cit., p. 21.

16 Newton, op. cit., p. 578.

17 Putnam, op. cit., p. 136.

18 Ibid.

19 Fukuyama, op. cit., p. 26.

20 Ibid.

21 Ibid.

22 S. Bok. *Lying*. London: Quartet Books Limited, 1978, p. 41.

23 K. Arrow. Uncertainty and the Welfare Economics of Medical Care. *American Economic Review*, 1963; III: 851–83.

24 R. La Porta et al. Trust in Large Organizations. *AEA Papers and Proceedings*, 1997; 87: 333–8.

25 Putnam, op. cit., p. 137.

26 I. Kawachi et al. Social Capital, Income Inequality and Morality. In *The Society and Population Health Reader: Income Inequality and Health*, Vol. 1, ed. I. Kawachi et al. New York: The New Press, 1999, p. 226.

27 Ibid.

28 Ibid.

29 Putnam, op. cit., p. 21.

30 R. Blendon et al. Understanding the Managed Care Backlash. *Health Affairs*, 1998; 17: 89.

31 L.J. Weiss and J. Blustein. Faithful Patients: The Effect of Long-Term Physician–Patient Relationships on the Costs and Use of Health Care by Older Americans. *American Journal of Public Health*, 1996; 86: 1742–7.

32 D. Mechanic. Changing Medical Organization and the Erosion of Trust. *Milbank Quarterly*, 1996; 74: 177; M.K. Wynia et al. Physician Manipulation of Reimbursement Rules for Patients: Between a Rock and a Hard Place. *Journal of the American Medical Association*, 2000; 238: 1858–65; P. Illingworth. Bluffing, Puffing, and Spinning in Managed-Care Organizations. *Journal of Medicine and Philosophy*, 2000; 25: 62–76.

33 J.R. Hampton et al. Relative Contributions of History-Taking, Physical Examination, and Laboratory Investigation to Diagnosis and Management of Medical Outpatients. *British Medical Journal*, 1975; 2: 486–98.

34 J.T. Hart. Two Paths for Medical Practice. *The Lancet*, 1992; 340: 772–5.

35 See, for example, J. Tudor Hart and P. Dieppe. Caring Effects. *The Lancet*, 1996; 347: 1606–8; J. Turner et al. The Importance of Placebo Effects in Pain Treatment and Research. *Journal of the American Medical Association*, 1994; 27: 1609–14.

36 M. Ahern and M. Hendryx. Social Capital and Trust in Providers. *Social Science and Medicine*, 2003; 57: 1195–1203.

37 Personal communication with Dr M. Hendryx, suggesting that this is consistent with their data, 19 March 2003.

38 Putnam, op. cit. p. 140; U.S.A. Today/CNN/Gallup Poll, 5–8 July 2002, as described in J. M. Jones. Poll Analyses: Americans Express Little Trust in CEOs of Large Corporations or Stockbrockers. *Gallup News Service*, 17 July 2002.

39 Comparative surveys show that physicians are among the most highly trusted professionals. For example, a 2002 Gallup Poll found that doctors are among the 10 most trusted professions, with 66 percent of those polled responding that most physicians can be trusted. (U.S.A. Today/CNN/Gallup Poll, op. cit.)

40 Mechanic, op. cit., pp. 171–89; L. Gilson et al. Trust and the Development of Health Care as a Social Institution. *Social Science and Medicine*, 2003; 65: 1453–68.

41 Putnam, op. cit., p. 137.

42 D. Mechanic and S. Meyer. Concepts of Trust Among Patients with Serious Illness. *Social Science and Medicine,* 2000; 51: 657–68.

43 Putnam, op. cit.

44 J.S. Coleman. Social Capital in the Creation of Human Capital. *American Journal of Sociology,* 1988; 94 (Suppl.): 116; S. Knack and P. Keefer. Does Social Capital Have an Economic Payoff? A Cross-Country Investigation. *Quarterly Journal of Economics,* 1997; 112(4): 1252–5.

45 L. Weiss, for example, found that faithful patients, those with long-term doctor–patient relationships, incurred somewhat lower medical costs. Long-term continuity of care may facilitate thick trust between doctors and patients and lower cost as a result. Weiss and Blustein, op. cit.

46 Putnam, op. cit., p. 117.

47 Ibid., p. 296; Coleman, op. cit., pp. 109–S113.

48 Ahern and Hendryx, op. cit.

49 Kawachi et al., op. cit.

50 Kawachi and Berkman, op. cit., p. 187. They suggest that, despite its status as a non-excludable public good, the poor, women, and African Americans may not have access to social capital because of residential segregation and other forms of discrimination.

51 I. Kawachi et al. Introduction. In Kawachi et al. (eds), *The Society and Population Health Reader: Income Inequality and Health,* Vol. 1, op. cit., pp. xx–xxi.

52 Putnam, op. cit., p. 19.

53 Ibid., p. 140.

54 Ibid.

55 U.S.A. Today/CNN/Gallup Poll, op. cit.

56 D. Mechanic. The Functions and Limitations of Trust in the Provision of Medical Care. *Journal of Health Politics and Law,* 1998; 23: 661–86.

57 Putnam, op. cit., p. 21.

58 E.H. Morreim. *Balancing Act: The New Medical Ethics of Medicine's New Economics.* Washington, DC: Georgetown University Press, 1995, p. 142.

59 Ibid.

60 A.A. Gawande et al. Does Dissatisfaction With Health Plans Stem From Having No Choices? *Health Affairs,* 1998; 17: 184–94; Kaiser Family Foundation. *Chartbook: Trends and Indicators in the Changing Health Care Marketplace,* May 2002.

61 J.S. Mill. *On Liberty.* Cambridge, UK: Hackett Publishing Company, 1978, p. 9.

62 This is an implication of Mill's well-recognized harm principle.

63 Mill, op. cit., p. 93.

64 Compare the interest in a low-trust doctor–patient relationship with the inter-
    est in divorce. Both probably lower social capital, yet the interest in being able
    to end a bad marriage is more important for individual well-being than is the
    interest in being able to maintain a low-trust relationship. I wish to thank
    W. Parmet for bringing this comparison to my attention.
65 Mill, op. cit., p. 9.
66 Ibid.
67 W. Frankena. *Ethics,* 2nd ed. New Jersey: Prentice Hall, 1973, p. 45.
68 Ibid.
69 J.S. Hause et al. Social Relationships and Health. In *The Society and Population
    Health Reader: Income Inequality and Health,* Vol. 1, op. cit., pp. 161–70.
70 See J. Stuart Mill. What utilitarianism is: In *Utilitarianism,* ed. O. Piest. Indiana:
    Bobbs-Merrill Educational Publishing, 1957.
71 Illingworth, op. cit.
72 Ahern and Hendryx, op. cit.
73 Gawande et al., op. cit., pp. 184–94.
74 I. Berlin. Two Concepts of Liberty. In *Liberalism and its Critics*, ed. M. Sandel.
    New York: University Press, 1984.
75 Putnam, op. cit., p. 414; Fukuyama, op. cit., p. 11.
76 Newton, op. cit., p. 582.
77 Putnam, op. cit.
78 M.G. Bloche and P. D. Jacobsen. The Supreme Court and Bedside Rationing.
    Journal of the American Medical Association, 2000; 284: 2776–9.
79 Kaiser Family Foundation, op. cit., p. 28.
80 D. Altman and L. Levitt. The Sad History of Health Care Cost Containment as
    Told in One Chart. *Health Affairs,* 23 January 2004, Web Exclusive W-83,
    pp. 1–2.
81 R. McNamara. Capitation for Cardiologists: Accepting Risk for Coronary
    Artery Disease Under Managed Care. *American Journal of Cardiology,* 1998;
    82: pp. 1178–82.
82 T. Maeder. Good Health is Just a Costly Way to Die. *Red Herring,* 1 September
    2000, pp. 55–60.
83 Ibid.

6 Law, its meaning, and its effect on social capital

The doctor–patient relationship has the potential to confer benefits on the community. Nonetheless, its ability to create trust and foster social capital has been impaired by some aggressively managed care. Although many of the cost containment mechanisms that managed plans use burden the doctor–patient relationship, these plans are not alone in imposing this burden on the community. Just as the doctor–patient relationship can either increase or decrease social capital, so too can the laws and policies that govern the health-care system and the community. Although public policy can, in general, affect social capital, in our discussion we will focus specifically on laws that inform health policy.[1] Some legal statements have discouraged the production of social capital indirectly by enabling managed care and directly by lowering social levels of trust. My analysis of some of the law relevant to managed care is intended to be illustrative rather than comprehensive and exhaustive. The point to be drawn from this discussion is that health plans are not alone in affecting the potential of the doctor–patient relationship to create social capital. Public policy has also played a role, as have employers.

Thus, any solution to the problems will require the cooperation of a number of legal and social institutions and organizations. I will look at three legal statements that have been important for the history of managed care and that 'speak to' social capital: (1) the Employment Retirement Income Security Act (ERISA), (2) the Supreme Court case, *Pegram v. Herdrich*,[2] and, for different reasons, (3) the professional practice standard. With the conceptual help of the expressive theory of law, I shall demonstrate that the legal statements under consideration have communicated meanings that are likely to discourage the production of social capital. This is a modest exploration. There are no doubt many laws that support the doctor–patient relationship and the trust it engenders, including fiduciary law and case law such as *Wickline v. State of California*.[3] More recently, the Supreme Court's decisions in *Rush Prudential HMO, Inc. v. Moran*[4] provided for a 'right' of independent review of medical disputes, and in *Kentucky Association of Health Plans, Inc. v. Miller, Commissioner, Kentucky Department of Insurance*[5] supported any willing provider laws against managed health plans. But this support for patients and their physicians has by no means been uniform.[6]

If there is a connection among law, policy, and social capital levels, we will need to think more creatively about the role social capital is to play in the policy and law we craft. Laws can only begin to protect and develop social capital if we are mindful of the need to do so. Failure to explicitly account for social capital will result in laws that depreciate our fund of social capital. Understanding the connection between law and social capital is a first step in this direction.

Expressive theories of law

The expressive theory of law can give us a framework for understanding the potential impact of the law on both the doctor–patient relationship and social capital. According to the expressive theory of law, in addition to directly controlling or facilitating conduct through contract, admonitions, and prohibitions, the law also serves an expressive function.[7] It communicates a social meaning, fashioning social norms. Indeed, much of the law's work can be achieved through these less coercive, indirect means.

Laws can be evaluated on the basis of how well they serve their expressive function. Cass Sunstein illustrates this point with the example of emissions trading.[8] One way that the law can control environmental pollution is through emissions trading systems that allow for the sale of emissions (rights to pollute), with the goal of eventual reduction in their numbers and the amount of pollution emitted. Sunstein points out that a number of people object to emissions trading on the grounds that '[it] may have damaging effects on social norms by making people see the environment as something without special claims to public protection.'[9] Some people would argue that negative expressive harms of this kind are in and of themselves enough to justify rejection of a law. But Sunstein believes, and I think rightly, that harmful expression will often coincide with other kinds of harms. In other words, if emissions trading does harbor serious expressive harms, these laws will also ultimately have bad consequences. In this way, the expressive and consequential purposes of the law can coincide. For Sunstein, legal statements that produce bad consequences should not be endorsed.[10]

Other laws, closer to the heart of bioethicists, also illustrate the social meaning conveyed by laws. For example, laws that affect how we value human life often evoke strong expressive meaning. Some of the debate around whether physician-assisted suicide should be legalized has to do with the impact of such laws on how we view persons and the sanctity of human life, much of it originating among disability-rights scholars.[11] Prior to this, similar concerns surfaced with the controversies over abortion and ending life-saving treatment.

Norm management is an important part of solving collective action problems. Sometimes the expressive function of a law can itself be the main reason for a change in behavior—as, for example, when a law is unaccompanied by enforcement. Typically people pick up after their dogs, even though such laws are rarely enforced, and potential violators are not always in a position to be seen by others. Once people have internalized the norms implicit in the law, actual monitoring may become unnecessary. In these cases, the expressive function of the law is doing all of the work. Being a responsible dog owner has become one of the values of good citizenship.

The law's expressive function can be served well or poorly. One way to measure the performance of the law's expressive function is in terms of how well it fits with other social norms and values. We have seen in previous chapters that trust and social capital are important for enhancing the values associated with citizenship and essential for individual and community welfare. Given this, it would be helpful to look at how laws relevant to managed care fare with respect to social capital. Laws that discourage trust and deplete social capital do not sit comfortably with other social values, such as our commitment to civic responsibility. When it becomes evident that our laws are adversely affecting our wherewithal to produce social capital, we may opt to create different kinds of laws. At the very least, we should fashion laws, mindful of their effect on social capital. Although law makes extensive use of enforcement mechanisms, such as the police, punishment, and the threat of punishment, it no doubt also relies heavily on social capital. Many people refrain from breaking the law because they realize that breaking the law can carry a cost to trust and social capital. In some respects, the breaking of a law can be viewed as a breach of trust.

ERISA: a window of opportunity

Most Americans receive their health care through their employers.[12] These benefits, including health insurance, are governed by the Employment Retirement Income Security Act (ERISA).[13] Despite the dependence of Americans on their employers for their health insurance, ERISA neither requires that employers give their employees insurance, nor does it specify the substantive benefits that need to be included in a health plan.[14] At the time of enactment, the stated purpose of ERISA was to protect employee pensions from abuse by those who invest and manage them.[15]

ERISA preempts state laws relating to employee benefits plans. Here the concern is with state laws that focus on the regulation of benefits plans.[16] Included as laws that relate to benefits plans are state laws that mandate particular benefits, but also state tort laws such as medical malpractise. Whether or not a state law is preempted depends on whether courts view it as 'relating to' a benefit plan. For example, state laws that regulate the business of insurance are 'saved' from preemption and thus states may indirectly regulate some plans under their 'right' to regulate the business of insurance. However, under the 'deemer' clause, employers who provide health benefits through plans that self-insure and assume the risks of insuring within the organization are able to sidestep state law regulating health insurance.[17] The prospect of avoiding the costly implications of some of these state laws has motivated many employers to self-insure.[18] In 1998, 50 percent of insured workers were enrolled in self-insured plans that were beyond the reach of such state insurance laws.[19]

When ERISA was enacted, the federal government had an interest in ensuring that organizations with offices in more than one state would only be subject to federal law and not to various and inconsistent state legislation. State laws that do not apply to ERISA self-funded plans include, for example, laws that mandate certain benefits and state tort and contract law.[20] Thus ERISA preempts state law, putting those plans beyond the reach of much state legislation. Subscribers who receive their health benefits from their employers in a self-insured plan do not have the protection of state regulation. Moreover, there is a dearth of federal regulation in this area.

In *McGann v. H&H Music Company*, McGann's health plan had provided for one million dollars worth of benefits over a lifetime. However, after McGann applied to receive benefits for the treatment of AIDS, his employer canceled the initial group insurance plan and switched to a new self-insured plan. Following this switch, the employer limited lifetime health benefits for AIDS treatment to $5,000. The federal and district courts found that, under ERISA, the company had the right to change the terms of the plan.[21] Additionally, in *Shaw v. Delta Airlines, Inc*, the Supreme Court said, 'ERISA does not mandate that employers provide any benefits, and does not itself proscribe discrimination in the provision of employee benefits.'[22]

Looked at through the lens of *McGann v. H&H Music Company*, health-care benefits appear to be a purely voluntary gift that employers give to employees.[23] ERISA, then, frustrates the ability of states to regulate health care and to ensure substantial benefits for needy and expensive patient populations. ERISA indirectly encourages labor and business to design inexpensive plans around healthy populations, leaving the unhealthy minority to fend for themselves.[24] Insofar as ERISA frustrates state efforts at health-care regulation, and mainly for reasons having little to do with the legislative intent of ERISA, it may be argued that it also frustrates democratic efforts at health-care reform. It impairs the state's ability to protect those it was intended to protect.

Pegram v. Herdrich

The Supreme Court case *Pegram v. Herdrich* provides another example of how social capital may be undermined by legal statements.[25] Cynthia Herdrich received her insurance through her husband's plan, Carle HMO, a physician-owned health-maintenance organization. As an employer-based plan, Carle HMO was governed by ERISA. Although Herdrich went to her Carle physician with an inflamed appendix, she was required to wait eight days for an ultrasound of her abdomen. Later her appendix ruptured; she developed peritonitis and required surgery. Herdrich charged that the HMO's end-of-the year bonus to physicians/administrators caused them to be excessively parsimonious in their care and in exercising their discretion as ERISA fiduciaries. Many health-policy scholars and bioethicists hoped the cost containment mechanisms of managed care would be challenged in this important Supreme Court case.[26] However, in what was perceived by some as a victory for managed care, the Justices cited the need for physician incentives in HMOs and longstanding congressional support for the rationing of HMOs. Specifically, the Court held that the 'mixed eligibility and treatment decisions made by an HMO, acting through its physician, were not fiduciary acts within the meaning of ERISA.'[27]

On one reading of *Pegram*, the Court seemed to affirm the 'legitimacy' of HMOs when it denied Cynthia Herdrich's claim. Commenting on its decision the Court stated, 'The fact is that for over 27 years the Congress of the United States has promoted the formation of HMO practices. The Health Maintenance Organization Act of 1973 "allowed the formation of HMOs that assume financial risks for the provision of health and services."'[28] The Court put the matter back in Congress's hands with the following invitation, 'if Congress wishes to restrict its approval of HMO practices to certain preferred forms, it may choose to do so.'[29] Recently, however, in *Cicio v. Vytra Health Care*,[30] the United States Court of Appeals for the Second Circuit in New York interpreted *Pegram* to have thrown 'cold water' on the reading of ERISA, according to which HMOs cannot be sued for their medical decisions. In *Cicio v. Vytra*, the court found that patients could sue HMOs and their medical directors for medical malpractice when they refuse to provide medically necessary care. It will be interesting to see whether the courts will follow in the recognition of patients' right to sue their ERISA plans for refusal to authorize medically necessary care.

Traditionally, the law functions both as a facilitator and a monitor of conduct. In the U.S., the right of consumers to sue medical professionals has contributed both to the maintaining of high standards of competency, as well as to negotiating an otherwise potentially harmful power imbalance. The same practical considerations that speak for a strong right to sue physicians also speak for a right to sue MCOs. Although it would be morally problematic to deny patients a full right to external review, it would be a mistake to assume that patient participation in such an adversarial process would contribute to our reservoir of social capital.[31] Many of the values that contribute to building trust and social capital, such as expressions of concern, cooperation, and a willingness to extend oneself without immediate reciprocation, are absent from the adversarial process.

To consider the impact of the 'legal statements' discussed in this chapter on social capital, we now need to look at their expressive function. Each of these 'statements' can potentially convey a number of meanings, some of which will vary with the context. My interest is in those meanings that speak to social relations, trust, and social capital. When we explore the expressive statements implicit in these legal statements, they seem to convey the message that when it comes to individual health, the law leaves individuals and communities to their own devices. In this way, laws that buttress managed care, such as ERISA, may contribute to the depletion of social capital and, in turn, to the benefits that we have come to associate with it.

Expressive content and social capital

Let us begin our brief exploration of some of the legal statements relevant to managed care with a consideration of the expressive content in ERISA. Health care in the U.S. primarily falls within the state's police powers, but can also fall under the *parens patriae* power.[32] Lawrence Gostin defines police power in the following way:[33]

> The inherent authority of the State . . . to enact laws and promulgate regulations to protect, preserve, and promote the health, safety, morals, and general welfare of the people. To achieve these communal benefits, the state retains the power to restrict, within federal and state constitutional limits, private interests—personal interests in autonomy, privacy, association, and liberty, as well as economic interests in freedom to contract and uses of property.

As this definition suggests, police powers are broad. Under the *parens patriae* power states have the duty to protect and care for individuals who cannot care for themselves, such as minors and the mentally disabled.[34] States have developed quite elaborate regulatory mechanisms toward the end of protecting the health of their community members, and include many of the state mandates that are preempted by ERISA.

The connection between the state's police power and its duty to protect the sick and vulnerable is inescapable. Laws that fall under police powers communicate the reassuring message that the state will care for those who fall within their scope. Thus, legal statements that reflect police and *parens patriae* powers convey many of the social meanings needed to build a large reservoir of social capital.

Many laws that fall within the state's police power are thus valuable sources of social capital. State mandated benefits, for example, express the concern of the state for the community and fall within the state's police powers. People who receive their insurance in ERISA-governed plans and are self-insured will not have the help of many of the state laws that protect other residents. They forfeit, often unwittingly, the protection afforded by those state rights when they opt for ERISA-based insurance. Moreover, they do not simply substitute federal protection for state protection. Since health care has not traditionally been within the scope of the federal government there is very little federal law in this area.[35]

Nor can it be argued that the state protections lost by those in ERISA self-insured plans are assumed by employers. Employers are first and foremost bound by fiduciary obligations to the organization and shareholders. They are mainly interested in their employees when they can take care of themselves—that is, when the employee will be a valuable member of the workplace. Moreover, as Marcia Angell and Jerome Kassirer point out, given the proclivity of American workers to move from job to job, the benefits from investing in the health of one's employees may seem to be just as likely to be realized by one's competitors as by the original employer.[36] Remember what happened to poor McGann when he tried to secure benefits for treatment of AIDS. His employer, H&H Music, switched to a less generous plan that would not include the expensive care McGann needed.[37] The question about what duties employers ought to assume directly is addressed in Chapter 7.

An employer's commitment to the health and welfare of his employees can be short-term and minimal. Although there are noted exceptions, employers are, for the most part, interested in healthy employees and healthy profits. Their interest is not in an employee's long-term health, nor in the harm that employees will feel in a trust-compromised doctor–patient relationship. Nor are they interested in the costs incurred by cost shifting as sick employees call upon relatives to care for them. This is not to say that there will not be times when employers will be more generous with health-care benefits, perhaps to reward loyal employees in flush times, or to attract promising employees in a particularly competitive job market.[38] But these benefits are negotiated. They rarely reflect concern, care, help, or the generalized reciprocity associated with social capital. They do not contain the ingredients that make up social capital. Indeed, in the wake of the tragedy at the World Trade Center on 9/11, in the midst of recession, many employees found their health benefits compromised.[39]

Considered as a legal statement, ERISA does not bode well for social capital. ERISA doesn't even require that employers provide employees with minimum health-care benefits. Considered in this light, ERISA may be interpreted to have all but abandoned its citizens. In some cases ERISA appears to have deprived employees of the protection afforded by state law and to leave it up to them to negotiate their benefits with their employers. This is not a particularly rational way to determine what health care people have access to since health itself has very little to do with an employee's marketability in the workforce. Moreover, many illnesses have a public dimension insofar as illness, whether or not it is contagious, affects other people. From a public welfare perspective it is arguably imprudent to leave the question of what health benefits people should have in the hands of organizations primarily motivated by profit.

ERISA leaves people, even the insured, to worry about whether, should they become sick and vulnerable, they will be able to receive the care they need. Some people will suffer unnecessarily because not being able to afford their portion of the employer-based insurance, they are uninsured. Other people will receive inadequate care. Still others will receive adequate care, but will worry that as the labor market changes, so will their benefits. Everyone will worry. As we saw in Chapter 5, the cultivation of social capital requires high levels of trust. It also requires the ingredients needed for an attitude of generalized reciprocity, including the willingness to forgo immediate reciprocation because of a belief in the goodwill of others. Generalized reciprocity depends on the existence of optimism based on trust in others, and it is incompatible with a world guided by the principle of 'for each his own.' It may be difficult for people who feel uncared for when they are sick to be optimistic about their future prospects and this, in turn, makes the cultivation of generalized reciprocity difficult. If people cannot be confident that they will receive the care they need from others when they are sick, vulnerable, and most needy, they have little reason to trust that others will act responsibly both with respect to themselves and others in the future. From the perspective of increasing our reservoir of social capital, the message conveyed by ERISA that the health of the community is dependent on the exigencies of employers, governed only by the minimalist requirements of ERISA, seems incompatible with the values that are at the heart of social capital.

Moreover, ERISA preemption of state law severely curtails the right and practice of patients to sue health plans for medical injuries.[40] Although patients in ERISA plans can sue their physicians for malpractice, some health-care plans cannot be sued despite their extensive influence on clinical decisions. In these cases, physicians may bear extensive liability for a patient's medical harm while the health plan (a co-decision maker) is insulated from liability because of ERISA preemption.[41] Recently, following *Dukes v. U.S. Healthcare Inc.* and its progeny, some significant chunks were cut out of ERISA preemption and its protection of health plans by way of a distinction drawn between the quality of care and the quantity of care.[42]

ERISA also limits the damages that plaintiffs can recover to the actual cost incurred for the benefit. Damages for pain and suffering and punitive damages, for example, are not available in disputes concerning ERISA plans. These limitations make it difficult for potential plaintiffs to find a willing lawyer and may, in turn, give health plans an incentive to deny care.[43] The right to legal recourse in the face of injury to one's physical and emotional well-being is among other things symbolic of full personhood in the U.S. In some respects being a rights holder is a measure of the extent of one's full engagement in the community. Children and prisoners do not, for example, enjoy full legal rights, and they are not seen by many as full members of the community.

Through ERISA preemption, the federal government has deprived aggrieved patients of an important moral right and has done so in deference to business interests. One message implicit in ERISA is that health care comes at the price of individual rights for those who purchase it from their employers. This is no small matter. The point is made nicely by Barry Furrow when he says, 'tort rules are more than a tax device, a crude source of economic deterrence of substandard behavior. Tort rules are moral beacons: They give voice to patients who have been patronized, ignored, actively manipulated at times, or cruelly treated by physicians.'[44] The right to sue those who are responsible for their harm gives patients social confirmation in their efforts to exact retribution for a medical harm. It provides them with public affirmation of the grievance they feel. In this way, lawsuits can be healing for patients. Nonetheless, the right to sue is a poor substitute for social capital. If anything this right comes into effect when social capital is low or has failed. It would be a mistake to treat the rights to sue and undertake an appeal as panacea to the problem of depleted levels of social capital. Many patients will be too sick to exercise these rights.

Greater understanding of the social message inherent in ERISA, especially as it is embedded in the current health-care system, can be gained by stepping out of this paradigm to briefly reflect on another very different one. Although international comparisons are difficult to make and are inevitably an oversimplification, they can serve as useful intuition pumps. Canadians have a system of universal access to health care. Although recent federal cutbacks have taken a toll on Canada's health-care system and contributed to its deterioration, the Canadian system is informed by a very different set of values than those that underlie the health-care system in the United States.[45] The Canadian health-care system, as stated in the preamble of the Canadian Health Act of 1983, is founded on five basic principles: (1) public administration, (2) comprehensiveness of medically necessary care, (3) universality, (4) portability, and (5) accessibility. The preamble to the Canadian Health Act states:[46]

> Canadians, through their system of insured health service have made outstanding progress in treating sickness and alleviating the consequences of disease and disability among all income groups . . . that continued access to quality health care without financial or other barriers will be critical to maintaining and improving the health and well-being of Canadians.

Looked at as a legal statement, the Canadian Health Act expresses the message that the federal government is committed to the care and well-being of Canadians. Furthermore, when the Act states that 'Canadians . . . have made outstanding progress in treating sickness', the implication is that fellow Canadians share a concern and responsibility for the welfare of all. Although comparing ERISA and the Canadian Health Act is a little like comparing apples and oranges, the comparison is nonetheless a useful one in the sense that ERISA governs the health insurance of most Americans, and the Canadian Health Act the health insurance of all Canadians. These provisions reflect the ethical, social, and political paradigm toward health care in their respective countries and influence the expressive potential of the law with respect to health care. The expressive content of Canada's Health Act would seem to be far more productive of social capital than ERISA. Even the Romanow Report, a recent critical evaluation of Canada's troubled health-care system, concluded with support for the principles underlying the system—'equity, fairness and solidarity'—and with the statement, 'Canadians view Medicare as a moral enterprise, not a business venture.'[47] Solidarity is at the heart of the Canadian system, reassuring Canadians that come what may, they will face individual challenges to health together. This approach has the wherewithal to purchase them considerable social capital.

Consider now the expressive content of the Supreme Court's decision in *Pegram v. Herdrich*. The Court's decision was complicated and no doubt sent mixed messages to, among others, legal scholars. Though many people view the decision as a triumph for managed care, still others see it as pro-patient. Gregg Bloche, for example, has the following to say about the *Herdrich* case:[48]

> The Supreme Court delivered the *coup de grace* last year in a case the managed care industry had thought it had won. The justices unanimously rejected an Illinois woman's federal suit against her HMO for its practice of rewarding doctors for withholding care. But in so doing, the High Court suggested that suits against health plans for denying care belong in state court.

Whether it was in fact a *coup de grace* or a victory for managed care will be determined in the future. Nonetheless, the Court did indicate approval of Congress' support for the incentives of managed medical care, and appears to have removed legal challenges to these incentives based on ERISA.[49] At one point, in footnote 8, the Court indicated that although the incentives themselves may be consistent with congressional intent, fiduciary duties may require that plan subscribers be informed about the presence of these incentives.[50] Put differently, it may be permissible to withhold treatment from patients provided that they are informed in advance. Again, it is difficult to know exactly how this will be interpreted, but one might suppose it reasonable to interpret it as the Court's support of liberty of choice, over their concern with the substantive welfare of the community.

According to the much-discussed footnote 8 of *Pegram v. Herdrich,* the Court implies that Herdrich's physician may have had an ERISA fiduciary duty to disclose the financial incentives.[51]

> The fraud claims in Herdrich's initial complaint, however, could be read to allege breach of fiduciary obligation to disclose physician incentives to limit care . . . Although we are not presented with the issue here, it could be argued that Carle is a fiduciary insofar as it has dis-

cretionary authority to administer the plan, and so it is obligated to disclose characteristics of the plan and of those who provide services to the plan, if that information affects beneficiaries' material interests.

Although duties of disclosure may be required by ERISA, they will do little to reinstate trust in the relationship between doctor and patient, at least not when the disclosure reveals interests at odds with the interests of patients. Disclosure may undermine trust created by the 'encapsulated interest' that we discussed in Chapter 3.[52] Although openness and honesty in general serve the interests of trust, when the disclosure reveals conflicts of interest, it may threaten trust. A duty to disclose financial incentives in the present context may put trust at greater risk since such disclosure will reveal to patients that their physicians are under a conflict of interest.[53] I am not advocating that we withhold this information from patients—but at the same time, let us not be deceived about what such disclosure will and will not achieve.[54]

Many of the problems associated with managed care have been attributed to the fact that ERISA-based self-insured plans are to some extent shielded from the usual legal recourse that patients have in the event of physician wrongdoing.[55] Consider this from the perspective of trust based on encapsulated interest. Recall that with respect to this kind of trust, patients are able to trust their physicians when they can see that it is in the interest of their physicians to behave in trustworthy ways. The right to sue may be one of the factors that permit people to take risks with their physicians and to place trust in them. Presumably, the physician/trustee will behave in certain ways in order to avoid being the object of a lawsuit. From the perspective of medical professionals, the prospect of legal suit by patients affects professional conduct and encourages behavior that warrants trust. It is not my intention to overstate this claim. Clearly there is room for reform of the tort system for medical injuries. My more modest claim is that having a legal right to sue for an injury may enable trust because it gives people an alternative in the face of disappointment and injury. The possibility of lawsuits and trust go hand in hand. There is no reason to believe that the same would not be true vis-à-vis patients and their health plans.

A right to sue a health plan is essential for patients. This is not to say that lawsuits are an effective way to build trust between doctor and patient. Nonetheless, health plans would probably be less inclined to adopt aggressive cost-cutting strategies that impair doctor–patient relationships if they could not do so with impunity.[56] We need to distinguish between building trust prospectively in the shadow of legal possibilities and the impact on individuals' levels of trust should they have to act on their right to sue. The former is trust building while the latter is likely to be trust diminishing.

We have looked briefly at how ERISA and *Pegram v. Herdrich* express meanings that discourage the creation and maintenance of social capital.

Legal statements that condone the use of financial incentives that may force patients to frequently change physicians, to haggle with providers, administrators, and appeals boards over benefits they need to save lives, or to spend less time with family and friends to access care, compromise our reservoir of social capital.[57] They do this in two ways. First, such legal statements facilitate the implementation of MCO practices that undermine trust and social capital. Second, they foster a moral paradigm that is inconsistent with the more community-oriented values we need to build a strong foundation of trust and social capital. Naturally, there is a concern that community members will treat each other with the same attitude of indifference to their welfare implicit in the legal statements at which we have looked.

The professional practice standard

A number of scholars and bioethicists have supported modifying the professional practice standard so that it would more accurately reflect the realities of health-care reimbursement.[58] As we saw in Chapter 4, the professional practice standard specifies one standard of care, though it can change from community to community. Under managed care, patients pay for levels of care from, for example, minimal benefits to full and comprehensive benefits.[59] That is, not all health plans provide sufficient benefits to meet the professional practice standard. It has been argued that it is unfair for physicians to be liable for providing one standard of care (the professional community standard), when health plans do not provide the same benefits in all cases.[60] It has also has been argued that as a matter of justice, patients are not entitled to more care than that for which they have paid.[61] If we look at the proposed revision of the professional practice standard as a legal statement, what message does it convey with respect to trust and social capital?

The professional practice standard is the standard of care used in tort law that determines what physicians' legal duties are to their patients. Malpractice requires (1) evidence of a recognized standard in the medical community and (2) evidence that the physician has negligently departed from that standard.[62] As with any negligence suit, the plaintiff must show that she has (3) suffered an injury, and that (4) the negligent behavior was the proximate cause of her injury.[63] On the professional practice standard, professionals are viewed as self-regulating; only other physicians are seen as knowledgeable enough about medicine to evaluate the performance of physicians. But the professional practice standard does more than specify a standard for malpractice. It also communicates certain norms, values, and symbols. And it can be looked at as a principle of resource allocation, according to which patients are entitled to receive from their physicians the same amount of health care as that received by other patients with the same illness living in the same area. Just as physicians are obligated to treat patients with a particular illness in the same way as other physicians treat their patients with that condition, so patients are entitled to the same treatment as other patients receive.

The professional practice standard does not transform the American health-care system into one that provides access to health care for all regardless of income, insurance status, race, or gender. Nonetheless, the professional practice standard produces, in principle, one standard of care. A physician's legal duty to a patient is identified, not by looking at what insurance the patient has, but by looking at what the patient needs and what other physicians do. According to this standard physicians are responsible for providing to patients the care that most physicians, practicing that specialty in that community would provide. Thus, the professional practice standard dictates the delivery of one standard of care to patients who come before the care of a physician.

Of course, insofar as physicians respond to managed-care incentives by modifying what they would typically do, health plans that manage care are, at the same time, changing the standard of care. In contrast, fee-for-service complemented the professional practice standard because it gave physicians the ability to access resources for their patients based primarily on professional judgment, regardless of the ability of particular patients to pay. In principle, when the professional practice standard was combined with fee-for-service, it produced one standard of care, at least for those with health insurance who were able to access the system. This is not to say that physicians provided patients with whatever they wanted, needed, or demanded. Physicians decided on a treatment plan based in part on available resources and, in part, on what other professionals were doing. By eroding the professional practice standard, managed care has, in turn, broken the values inherent in the professional practice standard.

Haavi Morreim has argued that the professional practice standard is an out-of-date concept, in need of modification. She proposes reshaping the legal standard for medical malpractice so that there are two standards, one of expertise, specifically the physician's medical expertise, and a second about health-care resources, which is about goods and services to lie in contract.[64] A number of legal questions can be raised about her proposal.[65] I will leave those questions for another time. Morreim's proposal for change can also be questioned on the basis of the ethics of a divided standard, and the expressive content inherent in such a change. She gives the following arguments in support of her proposed change. First, a divided standard of care would be fair to physicians in a way that the current standard is not. Second, a divided standard would acknowledge and legitimize unequal access to health care. Third, a divided standard of care would reflect the important role that patients can and should play in determining their access to health care.[66]

Let us review the arguments, beginning with the idea that physicians are treated unfairly when legally in malpractice they are required to provide one level of care to people of varying resources. Does the law place an undue moral burden on doctors? Surely, Morreim recognizes that the standard of care is fluid, responding in part to innovation, technology, and changes in reimbursement mechanisms. What becomes common practice in the medical community changes over time in response to these varying factors. Indeed, we can anticipate that in managed-care saturated areas, the standard of care will partially come to reflect what health plans are willing to pay for. That is, health plans will influence the standard of care. With respect to Morreim's first concern, there may not be as much of a disparity between the standard of care and what MCOs are willing to pay as she presupposes.

It will also be helpful to look at the standard of care through the eyes of physicians. From their point of view, the standard gives them the opportunity to be self-regulating and provides a useful way to monitor health plans and other health-care organizations. The standard of care can provide physicians with a tool that can be used to check health plans. It signals to physicians that they are the ones to determine the adequacy of benefits given certain illnesses. It serves as a check on the intrusion of the market.

Second, it would be a mistake to view unequal access to care as morally legitimate. Inequality in health care has always needed to be defended, but it certainly requires a defense in light of what we now know about the health and community benefits from social capital and equality in human relationships.[67] At any rate, the strongest argument in support of unequal access to health care is a liberty argument against the equal access argument. According to the latter, equal access to health care is unethical because it imposes too high a cost on individual liberty. This argument, however, is based on a narrow conception of negative liberty as freedom from interference. When liberty is thought of in positive terms as the liberty to do certain things, the liberty-based argument against equal access is less persuasive.[68]

Finally, the idea that a divided standard of care is preferable because it places the question of access to health care squarely on the shoulders of patients, is mistaken in light of what we know about the high cost of health insurance in this country and the difficulties many families experience trying to pay for it. Morreim has the following to say:[69]

> This obligation [to make their own decisions in matters of health and health care] . . . is a justice-based obligation of every agent to 'carry his own weight' in the moral community. One must not only fulfil the specific . . . duties such as keeping one's promises—but should also refrain from imposing unfair burdens on others.

Morreim goes on to say that this obligation extends not just to specific clinical choices, but also to choice of health-care plan. After all, she points out that all decisions involve trade-offs. If someone chooses minimal health benefits to save money for ski trips, we do not hurt him by honoring his decision. The physician who denies a patient a benefit in this situation, does not fail to meet her fiduciary duty, but merely respects the patient's free and voluntary choice.

This argument does not take into account the context in which people choose health insurance. To restate a point made often in this book, many people do not have a choice of plans, but are offered only one plan by their employer and many working Americans cannot afford to pay their portion of employer-based insurance—which during 1996 and 2001 vacillated between 27 and 30 percent of the cost of the plan.[70] That figure has remained relatively constant, hovering around 27 and 28 percent between 2002 and 2004.[71] We will discuss this further in the next as well as the last chapter.

It is wrong to assume that when people subscribe to a health plan they act freely. For Morreim, individual choice and individual property are key. For example, she states that we want, 'every agent to carry his own weight in the moral community.' She worries that '[p]atients cannot make responsible decisions so long as they think someone else pays the costs. They will never have the opportunity to evaluate the value of an intervention for themselves because they do not personally encounter the costs that are part of that value'.[72] At the same time, she is concerned that physicians are expected to 'commandeer other people's money and property on behalf of their patients.'[73]

Morreim is articulating a specific view of the moral life in which each individual is responsible for his own well-being and no one else's. Of course, if this is the prevailing ethical paradigm, it will lead to the belief not just that others are responsible only for themselves, but the converse, that they are responsible for no one other than themselves. This view, though fruitful in some respects, is bound to undermine the potential for trust, generalized reciprocity, and social capital. According to the conception of the 'good life' that Morreim articulates, people are unlikely to trust others because it is not really in the interest of others to be trustworthy since they are self-reliant. Similarly, the notion of generalized reciprocity has no place here. One can speculate that community levels of social capital would be low, as would the considerable benefits that trust and social capital confer upon patients, health-care organizations, and the community.

Social capital is the product of a world in which people do a little more than required, comfortable in the knowledge that they or someone else will benefit from a similar kindness in the future. In a world rich in social capital, each individual would carry his own weight and take a little bit of the weight off the shoulders of his neighbors. Unfortunately, the kind of moral community that Morreim sketches, in which each moral agent is responsible for himself, without expecting anything from others (especially not health care), is a world in which many of the benefits of trust and social capital are absent. Moreover, given the considerable health benefits associated with trust, social networks, and social capital, the costs of health care without social capital might well be greater than they need to be. As we continue to struggle with questions about society's obligation to provide health care to the community and balance the advantages and disadvantages of competing moral paradigms, we should be mindful of the moral resource of social capital.

Thinking about policy implications

I have suggested, using the expressive theory of law, that some legal statements convey messages that are inconsistent with the flourishing of trust and social capital. When crafting legal statements, such as ERISA, we need to be mindful of the potential for the loss in social capital that these statements may entail. As Oliver Wendell Holmes recognized about the common law, the law is fraught with varied considerations:[74]

> The life of the law has not been logic; it has been experience. The felt necessities of the time, the prevalent moral and political theories, intuitions of public policy, avowed or unconscious, even the prejudices that judges share with their fellow men, have a good deal more to do than the syllogism in determining the rules by which men should be governed.

Richard Daynard has argued, as have others in the law and public health movement, that consideration of the public's health needs to be among the canons that courts use in deciding cases.[75]

Daynard has identified a number of canons that the courts use, often to the disadvantage of public health. These are, for example, marketplace values, individual rights, strict constructionism, judicial administration, and common sense. Daynard believes that a concern for the public's health should be elevated to the same level as the concern for marketplace values and the other canons of judicial decision making. A similar tack could be taken with social capital. Judicial decision making needs to take social capital into account when cases are decided that can significantly affect social capital. Were courts to begin to take into account 'problems of public health' as a canonical consideration, surely social capital would be included. As we saw in Chapter 5, trust and social capital play an essential role in the public's health.

More specifically, federal law that imposes minimum requirements on health plans has the potential to foster trust within the doctor–patient relationship and is therefore to be encouraged, as is that version of the Patients' Bill of Rights that permits increased regulation of self-insured plans.[76] To leave self-insured plans in the hands of employers, with little protection from state law, will exacerbate the losses associated with diminished trust. Predictably, patients may feel betrayed not only by their physicians, their insurers, and their employers, but also by their state and federal governments. Moreover, the fear is that the messages conveyed by these legal statements will be first internalized by the community, then mirrored by them in their attitudes and conduct. Thus legal statements have the potential to affect our reservoir of trust and social capital. As we shall see in the next chapter, those who pay for health care, employers, also affect the kind of care people receive, and, in turn, trust and social capital.

Notes

1 L.F. Berkman. Social Networks and Health: The Bonds that Heal. In *The Society and Population Health Reader: A State and Community Perspective*. Vol. 2, ed. A.R. Tarlov and R. F. St Peter. New York: The Free Press, 2000, p. 272.
2 *Pegram v. Herdrich*, 530 U.S. 211 (2000).
3 *Wickline v. State of California*, 192 Cat. App 3d 1630 (1986).
4 *Rush Prudential HMO, Inc. v. Moran*, 536 U.S. 355 (2002).
5 *Kentucky Association of Health Plans, Inc. v. Miller, Commissioner, Kentucky Department of Insurance* 538 U.S. 329 (2003).
6 *Rush Prudential HMO, Inc. v. Moran*, op. cit.
7 C.R. Sunstein. On the Expressive Function of Law. 144 *University of Pennsylvania Law Review* vol. 2021, 1996, p. 2046.
8 Ibid.
9 Ibid.
10 Ibid., p. 2053.
11 A. Silvers. Protecting the Innocents: People with Disabilities and Physician-Assisted Dying. *Western Journal of Medicine*, 1997; 166: 407–9.
12 Kaiser Family Foundation. *Chartbook: Trends and Indicators in the Changing Health Care Marketplace*, 2004 Update, Exhibit 2.1.
13 The Employment Retirement Income Security Act of 1974 (ERISA), 1974.
14 W.E. Parmet. Regulation and Federalism: Legal Impediments to State Health Care Reform. *American Journal of Law and Medicine*, 1993; xix: 132–6.
15 H.R. Rep. No. 533, 93d Cong., 1st Sess. 3 reprinted in 1974 U.S.C.C.A.N. 4639, 4642.
16 P.D. Jacobsen. *Strangers in the Night*. New York: Oxford University Press, 2002, p. 133.
17 W.K. Mariner. Problems with Employer-Provided Health Insurance—The Employee Retirement Income Security Act and Health Insurance and Health Care Reform. *New England Journal of Medicine*, 1992; 327: 1683.
18 M.A. Chinba-Martine and T.A. Brennan. The Critical Role of ERISA in State Health Reform. *Health Affairs*, 1994; 13: 146.
19 G.A. Jenson and M.A. Morrisey. Employer Sponsored Health Insurance and Mandated Benefit Laws. *Milbank Quarterly*, 1999, 77: 426.
20 Mariner, op. cit.; *Implications of ERISA for Health Benefits and the Number of Self-Funded ERISA Plans*, EBRI Issue Brief #193, January 1998. Online, available at: <http://www.ebri.com> (accessed 2003).
21 *McGann v. H&H Music Company*, 742 F 392, S.D. Tex. 1990; *McGann v. H&H Music Company*, 946 F 2d 401, 5th Cir., 1991; cert. denied, *Greenberg v. H&H Music Company*, 61 U.S.L.W. 3355, 1992.
22 *Shaw v. Delta Airlines, Inc.*, 463 U.S. 85, 1983.
23 Although ERISA does not mandate specific substantial benefits, it does provide for specific fiduciary duties—such as duties of disclosure.
24 T.A. Brennan. An Ethical Perspective on Health Care Insurance Reform. *American Journal of Law and Medicine*, 1993; 19: 39–40.

25 *Pegram v. Herdrich*, op. cit.
26 L. R. Cohen et al. Brief of the Health Law, Policy and Ethics Scholars as Amici Curiae in Support of Respondent. *Pegram v. Herdrich*, No. 98–1949, 23–24, 20 December 1999.
27 *Pegram v. Herdrich*, 2000, op. cit.
28 Ibid.
29 Ibid.
30 *Cicio v. Vytra Health Care*, 321 F.3d 83 (2nd Cir. 2003).
31 A. Stone. *Law, Psychiatry and Morality*. Washington, DC: APA Press, 1984; H.J. Bursztajn. More Law and Less Protection: 'Critogenesis,' 'Legal Iatrogenesis' and Medical Decision Making. *Journal of Geriatric Psychiatry*, 1985; 18: 143–53.
32 For a discussion of the role of federal law in public health, see W.E. Parmet. After September 11: Rethinking Public Health Federalism. *Journal of Law, Medicine, and Ethics*, 2002; 30: 201–12; L.O. Gostin. *Public Health Law*. Berkeley, CA and New York: University of California Press and Milbank Fund, 2000, p. 47.
33 Ibid., p. 48.
34 Ibid., p. 51.
35 The following federal mandates supersede ERISA: The Mental Health Parity Act, 1996, New Born and Mothers Health Protection, 1996, Pregnancy Documentation Act, 1978, Consolidated Omnibus Budget Reconstruction Act (1985, COBRA), Health Insurance Portability and Accountability Act (HIPAA), 1996.
36 M. Angell and J.P. Kassirer. Quality and the Medical Marketplace—Following Elephants. *New England Journal of Medicine*, 1996; 335: 883–5.
37 *McGann v. H&H Music Company*, op. cit.
38 P. Fronstin. *Employment-Based Health Benefits*, EBRI Issue Brief # 233, May 2001. Online, available at: <http://www.ebri.com> (accessed 2003).
39 M. Simmons. For Newly Jobless, Insurance Options are Few. *New York Times*, Final Edition, 18 December 2001, Sec. FO1.
40 *Dukes v. U.S. Healthcare Inc.*, 57 F. 3d 350 (3d Cir. 1995) cert demand 530 U.S. 1242, 1995; *Bauman v. U.S. Healthcare, Inc.* (In Re U.S. Healthcare) 193 F. 3d 151 (3d Cir. 199), 530 U.S. 1242 (2000); *Lazorko v. Pennsylvania Hospital*, 237 F. 3d 242 (3d Cir.), 2000.
41 P. Jacobsen and S. Pomfret. ERISA Litigation and Physician Autonomy. *Journal of the American Medical Association*, 2000; 283: 921–6.
42 *Dukes v. U.S. Healthcare, Inc.*, 57 F. 3d 350 (3rd 350) (3rd civ. 1995); see also *Herrera v. Lovelace Health Systems, Inc.*, 35 F. Supp. 2d 1327 (D.M.N. 1999); *Crum v. Health Alliance-Midwest, Inc.*, 47 F. Supp. 2d 1013 (C.D. Ill. 1999); *Tufino v. NY Hotel and Motel Trades Council*, 646 NY S. 2d 799 (A.D. 1 Dept. 1996).
43 K. Polzer and P. Butler. Employee Health Plan Protections Under ERISA. *Health Affairs*, 1997; 16: 93–102.
44 B. Furrow. The Problem of Medical Misadventures: A Review of E. Haavi Morreim's Holding Health Care Accountable. *Journal of Law, Medicine, and Ethics*, 2001; 29: 381–95.
45 J.K. Iglehart. Revisiting the Canadian Healthcare System. *New England Journal of Medicine*, 2000; 342: 2007.
46 Preamble of Canada Health Act, R.S.C. 1985, c. C-6, Preamble.
47 R.J. Romanow. A Message to Canadians. In *Building on Values: The Future of Health Care in Canada (Final Report of the Commission on the Future of Health Care in Canada)*, November 2002.
48 Gregg Bloche, op. cit.

49 Jacobsen, op. cit., pp. 164–5.
50 *Pegram v. Herdrich*, 2000, op. cit.
51 Ibid.
52 D. Mechanic. Models of Rationing: Professional Judgment and the Rationing of Medical Care, 140 *University of Pennsylvania Law Review* 1713, May 1992.
53 Ibid.
54 S. Rosenbaum comments on a recent study showing that only about one third of appeals were for medical necessity, suggesting that this might be evidence of the extent to which members feel it is futile to appeal. S. Rosenbaum. Managed Care and Patients' Rights (Editorial). *Journal of the American Medical Association*, 2003; 289: 906–7; D.M. Studdert and C. Roan Gresenz. Enrollee Appeals of Preservice Coverage Denials at 2 Health Maintenance Organizations. *Journal of the American Medical Association*, 2003; 289: 864–70.
55 Jacobsen, op. cit., pp. 125–51.
56 Jacobsen and Pomfret, op. cit.
57 Haggling with Health Care Providers about their Prices Likely to Increase Sharply as Out-of-Pocket Costs Rise. H. Taylor and R. Leitman, eds., *Harris Interactive Healthcare News*, 2002; 2(5). Available at: http://www.harris interactive.com/news/newsletters_healthcare.asp
58 E.H. Morreim. *Holding Health Care Accountable*. New York: Oxford University Press, 2001.
59 It might be objected that it is wrong to attribute the presence of different levels of care to 'managed care.' Rather, some might maintain that this is a function of market medicine. However, by shifting the risk of treatment decisions from the insurer to the physician, managed-care plans can impose a burden on physicians who treat patients according to the professional practise standard—especially when the cost of doing so is high. Thus managing care can change physician behavior and eventually the standard of care itself.
60 E.H. Morreim. *Balancing Act: The New Medical Ethics of Medicine's New Economics*. Washington, DC: Georgetown University Press, 1995.
61 See E.H. Morreim. *Holding Health Care Accountable*, op. cit.
62 See *Davis v. Virginia R.R. Co.*, 361 U.S. 354, 357, 1960.
63 W. Prosser & W. Keeton. *Prosser and Keeton on the Law of Torts*, 5th edn. St Paul, Minn.: West Publishing Company, 1984, pp. 164–51.
64 E.H. Morreim. Medicare Meets Resource Limits: Restructuring the Legal Standard of Care, 59 *University of Pittsburgh Law Review* Vol. 1, 1997, p. 28.
65 See M. Hall. Healthcare Cost Containment and the Stratification of Malpractice Law. *Jurimetrics*, 1990; 30: 501–9.
66 E.H. Morreim. *Balancing Act: The New Medical Ethics of Medicine's New Economics*, op. cit., pp. 116–17.
67 Berkman, op. cit., pp. 259–77; L.F. Berkman. The Role of Social Relations in Health Promotion. In *The Society and Population Health Reader: Income Inequality and Health*. Vol. 1, ed. I. Kawachi et al. New York: New Press, 1999, pp. 171–83.
68 I. Berlin. Two Concepts of Liberty. In *Liberalism and Its Critics*, ed. M. Sandel. New York: NYU Press, 1984.
69 E.H. Morreim. *Balancing Act: The New Medical Ethics of Medicine's New Economics*, op. cit.
70 E. O'Brien and J. Feder. Employment-Based Coverage and its Decline: The Growing Plight of Low-Wage Workers. Prepared for the Kaiser Commission on Medicaid and the Uninsured. Washington, DC: Henry J. Kaiser Foundation, May 1999; Kaiser Family Foundation. *Chartbook: Trends and Indicators in the Changing Health Care Marketplace*, May 2002, p. 30.

71 Kaiser Family Foundation/Health Research and Educational Trust. *Employer Health Benefits 2004 Annual Survey,* September 2004, Chart #5.
72 E.H. Morreim. Redefining Quality by Reassigning Responsibility. *American Journal of Law and Medicine,* 1994; 20: 97.
73 Ibid., p. 89.
74 O.W. Holmes. *The Common Law.* Cambridge: Belknap Press, 1967. As quoted in R. Daynard. Regulating Tobacco: The Need for a Public Health Judicial Decision-Making Canon. *Journal of Law, Medicine and Ethics,* 2002; 30: 281–9.
75 Daynard, op. cit.
76 For a discussion of mandates, see Jenson and Morrisey, op. cit., pp. 425–59.

7 Employer leadership in the era of workplace rationing

Recent figures show that more than 175 million Americans have job-based health insurance.[1] Thus, employers have considerable influence over the health of their employees, the nature and quality of the health-care system in the United States, and the levels of trust and social capital available to individuals and the community. Despite the magnitude of their influence, because of ERISA they have been relatively free from regulation with respect to the specific substantive benefits they offer their employees. As we saw in the last chapter, ERISA gives employers enormous discretion to decide what substantive benefits they include in employer health plans.[2] But the decisions that employers make when they choose benefits for their employees are as much rationing decisions in need of ethical analysis as are the rationing decisions that are made at the bedside by physicians, patients, and their families. Moreover, even strong discretion, of the kind employers have, is subject to ethical standards. In view of what is at stake here, including the health of individuals and our reservoir of social capital, only the highest ethical standards are appropriate.

In this chapter I will maintain that it is reasonable to view employers as proxy decision-makers for their employees. As such, they should inform their decision making about employee health benefits on the basis of traditional proxy criteria, either (1) substituted judgment or (2) a modified version of the best-interest-of-the-patient test, namely, the best-interest-of-the-employee. When the question of what health benefits employees should be offered is considered in light of these criteria, many of the cost-saving practices recently used by employers, such as offering only one plan, will be seen as morally problematic. I further argue that for consequentialist and fairness reasons, employers have a duty to offer health plans that foster a trust-rich doctor–patient relationship.

Although ERISA and court interpretations of ERISA suggest that it is up to employers what benefits they give, or whether they give benefits at all, when we look at cross-disciplinary explanations of why business provides health-care benefits, a rather more complicated picture arises. Employers give a number of reasons for giving generous health-care benefits to their employees. Hefty benefits packages are seen as a way to avoid unionization.[3]

As unions became more common, businesses made greater efforts to increase employee satisfaction.[4] From an economic perspective, benefits are a form of compensation that employers use to attract good employees.[5] When we take these various explanations into account, the idea that benefits are best characterized as a gift seems implausible. For the most part, gifts are only given in the absence of a bargained-for exchange. Health benefits, on the other hand, are viewed as compensation. If these benefits are more than the supererogatory gifts of employers to employees, then it is certainly reasonable to assume that employers are bound by certain moral standards and obligations with respect to them.[6]

Starting with clinical ethics

Troyen Brennan has suggested that the way to determine an organizational ethic in the era of managed care is by way of a bottom-up approach in which institutional allocative decisions reflect the values that control the clinical setting.[7] This approach has the advantage of ensuring some consistency between allocative decisions and the values of clinical ethics. Brennan identifies three fundamental values of traditional medical ethics. First, 'that the health care provider be committed to the patient as a person of immeasurable value.'[8] Second, that 'institutions of medical care should support the morality of the doctor–patient relationship.'[9] In particular, Brennan states that health care policy should reflect the traditional commitment of medical ethics to altruism and selflessness.[10] Third, members of the provider community must see their actions as protecting one another and must be willing to act as a group when economic considerations hamper the care of particular patients.[11] Although Brennan seems to have this framework in mind as a guide to health-policy makers, it can also be a useful guide for employers who are making allocative decisions when they choose health-care benefits for their employees. Employers can fruitfully draw on the idea that the ethics of the doctor–patient relationship needs to inform their allocative decision-making.

A first step in this direction is to understand an employer's decision to choose certain employee benefits as proxy decision making. Marcia Angell and Jerome Kassirer have taken just this position. 'No longer do employers simply pay the bills; they now determine the details of the benefit package and its limitations. The doctor–patient dyad has been replaced by the health plan–employer dyad.'[12] By structuring the benefits packages that are available to employees, and often offering no more than one plan, employers determine the nature and quality of health care that their employees receive. Employers are torn between meeting their assumed responsibility to employees to provide health insurance and meeting their fiduciary duties to their shareholders to the organization to maximize profits. I shall provide reasons for balancing these conflicting duties in favor of employees. These reasons are two-fold, having to do both with the role of a proxy and with the potential to produce social capital.

Although the choice of health plans is complex, given the extent of the influence employers have over the choice of plan, it makes sense to view employers as proxy decision-makers for their employees. This is especially the case in self-funded employer plans, which are exempt under ERISA from many state mandates and other forms of state regulation. Robert Kuttner believes that, although it was once reasonable for employers to serve this proxy function, it no longer is.[13] But Kuttner's pessimistic conclusion would only follow if it were impossible to construct criteria that employers cum proxy decision-makers could use in designing health-benefits packages. Brennan's suggestions are instructive here. That is, we can look at clinical ethics, itself, to see what principles guide proxy decision making and apply them to employer decision making.

Employers cum proxy decision-makers

Typically, a proxy is 'a person who is substituted . . . by another to represent him and act for him. . . . Depending on the context, a proxy may also refer to the grant of authority itself. . .'.[14] Thus proxies make decisions for other people. The proxy most familiar to medical ethics is the proxy who makes treatment decisions for patients who cannot make those decisions for themselves, often end-of-life decisions.[15] Although in their capacity as subscribers to a plan, employees ultimately endorse a particular plan (that is, they subscribe to it), employers often determine precisely what that decision will be when they frame the options available to employees. This is especially so when employers offer only one plan.[16]

Before turning to a discussion of the criteria proxy decision-makers use in the clinical context, I want to set out the argument for viewing employers as proxies. Two basic features can be said to characterize proxy decision-makers. First, a proxy makes a decision on behalf of someone else. Second, those for whom the decision is made must, at the time the decision is made, have relatively little to say about the decision (though on substituted judgment their influence may inform the decision at an earlier time.) These features are present when employers decide on health benefits. Consider the following.

First, employers determine the nature and quality of health care for their employees by crafting specific benefits options. For example, since the 1980s, when employers became concerned with the increasing rate of inflation in health-insurance premiums, they took steps to contain health-care costs. The cost of providing employees with health care jumped in 1988 to 8.9 percent of wages and salaries, up from 2.2 percent in 1965. Some people viewed this escalation as responsible for putting the U.S. at a competitive disadvantage in the international business arena.[17] In the wake of the most recent recession, employers and health plans together continue to fashion new and increasingly cost-effective approaches to insuring employees.[18]

One way that employers responded to this increase in the cost of health care was to direct their employees into HMOs. In 1985 only 10 million Americans were enrolled in HMOs, while in 1996 that number had reached 50 million. Up until very recently (spring 2002), and in the shadow of the backlash against managed care, there has been a decline in employee enrollment in strict HMOs and an increase in enrollment in more flexible forms of managed care.[19] As of 2004, 55 percent of covered workers were enrolled in preferred provider plans (PPOs), up from 21 percent in 1993.[20] Some believe that this shift reflects dissatisfaction with strictly managed care. Premiums also increased by 13.9 percent from the spring of 2002 to the spring of 2003,[21] the largest increase in the cost of health insurance since 1989.[22] Much of the increase in the cost of health insurance was borne by employees. In the post 9/11 weak economy, the demand for workers declined, as did employers' incentive to entice employees with generous benefits packages. Employees experienced a 27 percent increase in the cost of single coverage in 2002; family coverage increased 16 percent from 2001 to 2002.[23] Since then, the increase in premiums has slowed. In 2004, the cost of single coverage increased by 7.7 percent, while family coverage increased by only 12.3 percent between 2003 and 2004.[24] Not surprisingly, the percentage of employers offering 'free' health insurance also declined.[25]

Employees also experienced significant increases at the time that they received services in the way of increased co-payments and deductibles.[26] Indeed, these increases have led some workers, such as those working at the General Electric Co., to go on strike.[27] Moreover, there does not appear to be an end in sight to escalating health-care costs for employers. In 2004, premium costs actually rose by 11.2 percent.[28] Although this increase is lower than the 13.9 percent of 2003, it is still in the range of double digit growth.[29] Even if the growth in the cost premiums stabilizes or declines, employees appear to be experiencing an increase in out-of-pocket spending on health care.[30]

The original shift into HMOs was a result of employer policies, including providing employees with only one plan, an HMO, or adopting a fixed-contribution method whereby cost conscious employees went with the cheapest (usually an HMO) plan available. Boeing, for example, offered its employees five plans from which to choose, including a traditional indemnity plan, but gave financial awards to workers who switched from the indemnity plan to managed care and remained with managed care.[31] These kinds of financial incentives would not encourage employees to undertake careful and comprehensive decisions about their health-care plans. From an ethics perspective, offering employees a choice of plans should enhance their self-determination and ensure that the choice of plan reflects their needs and wishes. However, encouraging them to choose one kind of plan over another with attractive financial incentives only undermines their wherewithal to choose thoughtfully. Given the tendency of subscribers to choose a plan primarily on the basis of price, and already disadvantaged by the general uncertainty about their health, such incentives detract from the potential for autonomous choice. Moreover, since the incentives will weigh more heavily for those employees with lower income, it will also detract from an equitable distribution of the benefits. When employers use financial incentives of this kind, they undermine the credibility of claims asserting that subscribers voluntarily choose to be managed.[32]

Employers also controlled costs by creating purchasing coalitions. By 1995, 8,000 employers had joined employer health coalitions.[33] The purchasing power of these coalitions allowed them to increase their negotiating power with HMOs and to secure a better deal. Purchasing coalitions retained the ability to drop pricey HMOs,[34] the threat of which influenced the behavior of HMOs. In addition, these coalitions turned to direct contracting with health-care providers, hospitals, and physicians. In this way, employers have gradually acquired the power to influence health-care organizations and the health benefits of their employees.

Large purchasers of this kind are closely involved with benefit design, often relying on consultants for technical expertise.[35] They have assumed the roles that were previously undertaken by health plans. One of the main coalitions, the Pacific Business Group on Health (PBGH) designs a standardized package and negotiates for 21 companies (400 beneficiaries).[36] The California Public Employees Retirement system negotiates with 11 HMOs for a standard benefit package on behalf of one million beneficiaries.[37] One reason organizations tailor their own packages is that, if they self-insure, ERISA exempts them from state laws.[38] Given the degree of employer participation in benefits design, it is reasonable to regard employers as proxy decision-makers for employees.[39]

Second, employees have relatively little influence over the health-care benefits they receive. To the extent that subscribers freely and voluntarily choose their health plans, employers arguably do not. In turn, the less involved employers are with plan design, the less they would qualify as proxies. But the results from surveys suggest that employees frequently do not exercise much choice over their health plans. Gawande et al. found in their survey that 42 percent of insured respondents were given no choice of health plan when they enrolled.[40] Of those who reported having choice, one in five stated that there was not enough variety among the options.[41] Thirty-one percent of adults surveyed reported being forced by their employer to change their plans between 1992 and 1997.[42] This survey also indicated that people with low income were disproportionately represented among those with no choice.[43] Given the absence of choice for many employees, combined with inadequate choice for others, the view that employers function as proxy decision-makers is buttressed. At least from their perspective, employees do not choose their benefits.

Employers have assumed an increasingly significant role in determining health benefits in part because labor has been less influential in these areas than in the past. Although historically labor played an important role in securing insurance for the American workforce,[44] its effectiveness in bargaining over health-care benefits has since waned. This can, in part, be attributed to relatively low employee participation in unions. In 2002, only 13.2 percent of wage and salary workers were members of unions.[45] Following Fox and Shaffer, Rosner and Markowitz argue that labor forfeited control over health benefits in exchange for greater access to health care for employers.[46] This trend was only exacerbated by the rise of managed care. 'Both the creation of management-controlled HMOs . . . which were completely unaccountable to the labor movement, and the extraordinary rise in costs, underscored the distance between the broad population of working people and the system that ostensibly offered them care.'[47] Moreover, even when unions are active in negotiating with employers about health plans, their negotiations may be ineffective. This was the experience reported by C. Montagne, a faculty representative on a benefits negotiations committee with a university administration.[48] The state of the labor market is of greater influence in determining what benefits employees receive: richer benefits in a tight labor market and poorer benefits in a loose market. Simply put, employers need to offer generous health benefits, among other things, in a tight market if they are to remain competitive.[49]

In the medical context, proxies decide on the basis of one of two criteria.[50] These are (1) substituted judgment and (2) the best interest of the patient. In the first, a proxy chooses a treatment option based on what she knows the patient would want, given what is known about the patient's desires, preferences, and values.[51] In the second, the proxy tries to determine what will actually be in the best interest of the patient from an objective point of view.[52] Sometimes what will be in the best interest of the patient coincides with what the patient would want, but not necessarily. Importantly, both of these criteria put the interests of the person for whom the decision is made first—whether those interests are viewed objectively or subjectively.

It might be argued that from the perspective of employers the focus on employees' medical interests is too narrow. Medical interests, after all, are potentially infinite and pursuit of them could put an organization in financial distress. This point needs to be taken seriously. But it is surely possible to balance the best interest of employees with the financial health of an organization. It may be that Brennan's considerations should be invoked here and that limits on the pursuit of the best medical interest of the employee can be set, provided that they respect the ethics of the doctor–patient relationship. Let us look at what both of these criteria imply for employer-based health benefits.

Implementing substituted judgment

Consider substituted judgment. Roughly, substituted judgment tells us that decisions should be made on the basis of what an individual would want. It takes seriously the value of autonomy, by claiming that the wishes of the person on behalf of whom the decision is made are what count. If we were to argue that employers should guide their decisions about their employees' health-care benefits on the basis of substituted judgment, then in order to accommodate individual preferences, they should opt for health benefits that leave as much open as possible to individuals to decide. Choice figures prominently among the health values of Americans. These findings have been repeated in other research venues.[53]

Donelan et al. conducted an international survey in which they questioned people about their concerns with health care. One in four Americans surveyed indicated having experienced difficulty securing medical care for either themselves or their family. The problems were largely attributed to finances or inadequate insurance.[54] The survey also found that people with traditional indemnity insurance were more likely to rate their physicians and medical care as excellent, whereas HMOs were a highly significant predictor of lower-quality ratings.[55] These findings speak to the question of how employers might implement substituted judgment.

Choice figures prominently among the features that subscribers value in a health-care plan. This can be inferred from the unhappiness elicited from subscribers who did not have choice. In the Gawande and Blendon survey, respondents were much less happy with their health plans when they did not choose them. This was even more pronounced when a care plan was one that could be described as heavily-managed care.[56] Subscribers appear to value having more than one plan to choose from and having real variation within those plans.[57] Enthoven and others found that consumer satisfaction would be greatly increased if employees were given the choice of plans that included a wide access plan such as fee-for-service, at a similar out-of-pocket premium cost.[58]

A relatively recent survey undertaken jointly by the Kaiser Family Foundation and Harvard School of Public Health found that Americans are growing ever more dissatisfied with managed care. In 1997, only 21 percent of Americans said that managed care was doing a bad job. By 2001, that figure had almost doubled to 39 percent. Still, 62 percent of Americans are satisfied with their health plans. However, people enrolled in strict managed care plans are less satisfied (58 percent) than those in loosely-managed-plans (63 percent), or traditional plans (74 percent). Nonetheless, although people are satisfied with their health plans, 24 percent are very worried that, if they become sick, their health plans will be more concerned about saving money than providing them with the best treatment, and 32 percent said that they were somewhat worried. People in strictly managed care were more worried than those in other plans (67 percent).[59]

A study done by Grumbach et al. is specific about some of the details of patient preferences. These researchers found that patients put a high value on their primary care physicians (PCP) both to integrate their care and to participate in decisions about referrals to specialists. They also found that patients wanted access to specialists when they believed they needed them and that a 'noteworthy' number believe that their primary care physician was an impediment to a specialist. The study found that patients viewing their PCP as an impediment to specialists was among the strongest predictor of low trust, confidence, and satisfaction ratings.[60]

The backlash against managed care can also serve as a clue to what subscribers want and don't want.[61] This backlash has taken the form of a public outcry in the media, grassroots mobilization, and the passage of legislation regulating managed care in almost every state across the country.[62] Grassroots responses to managed care have shown that people object to many of the economic incentives that MCOs use to contain costs. Blendon et al. undertook a study aimed at trying to understand this backlash. They report that a majority of those surveyed believe that sick patients will not receive the care that they need in managed care.[63] In a poll asking respondents to rank the importance of factors in choosing a health plan, they ranked the following in order of importance: (1) how well the plan cares for the sick, (2) cost to patients, (3) range of benefits, and (4) whether a person's doctors were in the plan. Then they indicated a preference for (5) a wide choice of doctors and (6) inclusion of one's preferred hospital in the plan. Finally, a preference for (7) whether the plan has been accredited, was indicated.[64] These rankings echo concern about the adequacy of care and choice, and suggest the importance of continuity of care for subscribers.

On the basis of studies showing that trust is important for the doctor–patient relationship and for the full therapeutic benefits of the relationship, we can infer that patients want a high-trust doctor–patient relationship.[65] Given the importance patients place on choice of doctor and having their own doctor, and the decline in patient trust when PCPs interfere with referrals in a plan, a substituted judgment approach should also be concerned with the quality of the doctor–patient relationships made possible by different kinds of health plans. That is, employers need to ensure not only that patients are able to choose their own doctors, but that those physicians are able to care for patients in a way that encourages trust. Plans that facilitate choice of physician and the ability of patients to continue with their own physician, but then modify physician behavior dramatically through financial incentives, are ultimately not respecting patient wishes.

Surprisingly, there is some evidence that, when subscribers purchase health insurance, they appear to be motivated primarily by price considerations such that they respond to small cost differentials. For example, at American Express, HMO enrollment jumped from 33 to 62 percent over two years following a fixed contribution policy.[66] Were we, for the purpose of implementing substituted judgment, to take what employees do as a signal of what they want, we might be led to conclude that subscribers want only the least expensive insurance. But actions are not a decisive indicator of wants. If actions can be accounted for by other reasonable explanations then they needn't be determinative. As I have shown, there is adequate survey material available to make reasonable inferences about what it is that patients value in their medical care and in turn from a health-care plan.

A counterargument to the view that employers should look to employee preferences in designing plans is that the potential set of employee preferences is much greater than what employers can be expected to provide. Arguably, however, our expectations of employers are determined at least partially by our understanding of the purpose such benefits serve for employers. The standard economic explanation for health benefits is worker demand, combined with the need of employers to attract good employees.[67] If this is an accurate account, then it makes sense for employers to provide *only* the amount of benefits that they can extend back to employees in the form of lower wages or as needed to attract employees. But what if this is not an accurate picture or is only part of the story?

Ellen O'Brien makes a business case for employee health benefits. O'Brien believes that part of the reason that employers are willing to act as employees' agents with respect to health insurance is employee preference.[68] However, she also believes that it makes good *business* sense for employers to do so. For one thing, health insurance provides employers with economic value because employees can be more productive when they are healthy. She points out that although the data are inconclusive, 'When employers factor in the indirect costs—such as those for replacement workers, overtime premiums, productivity losses due to unscheduled work absences, and productivity . . .—the cost burden is quite large' and 'frequently surpassed employers' direct expenditures on health benefits.'[69] If this is so, then employers may benefit financially from meeting the preferences of employees with respect to health plans. Thus it may be profitable for employers to provide employees with health insurance. If this is the purpose for employer-provided health benefits, then a different criterion for determining what benefits to offer emerges.[70] Employers can be more expansive in the benefits they offer employees because these benefits may in the end contribute to increased profits.

I have suggested how employers might identify subscriber wants for the purpose of implementing substituted judgment. Of course, some people would challenge the appropriateness of substituted judgment on the grounds that since subscribers are themselves competent decision-makers and are available, they should be consulted individually. Given this, there is no reason to invoke substituted judgment at all. I disagree. Employees have been consulted indirectly by way of the various surveys that have been undertaken, and they can be canvassed directly. Nonetheless, there is evidence that many people do not understand the complexity of their plans, even when informed.[71] As I suggested earlier in this chapter, employees have not in the recent past been effective negotiators in the area of health benefits, either directly or indirectly through labor organizations. But more to the point, substituted judgment is important because it tells us whose 'wants' count. In the case at hand, it instructs us to look at the preferences of employees.

Best-interest-of-the-employee test

Although there are important questions to be asked about how we determine what is in the best interest of the employee, we need to begin by identifying what sort of interests will qualify. When a proxy makes a decision about employee health care, the kinds of interests at issue are for the most part the medical interests of the employee. Given what we know about the health benefits to be had from trust, social relations, and social capital, 'medical' should be construed broadly. Moreover, it should be underscored that it is the employees' interests that count. The interests of others, such as stockholders, are less relevant to this calculation. As with substituted judgment, the point of a best-interest test is to specify that it is the interests of the designated that count and not someone else's. This is most clearly seen, for example, with the best-interest-of-the-child test that is used in family law. Although there may be important questions concerning how 'best medical interest' is to be identified, some interests are uncontroversial. All things considered, it is in the interest of employees to have health insurance as opposed to not having it.

Employer cost shifting and the failure to meet proxy criteria

Given recent trends in employer-based insurance, it would appear that employers have not adequately informed their decision making on the basis of either substituted judgment or the best-interest-of-the-employee test. As employers successfully stemmed the rising cost of health care that was encountered in the 1980s (even if only briefly), the number of employees without health insurance rose substantially.[72] In 1987, 69.2 percent of employees secured their health insurance from their employers.[73] Between 2000 and 2001 the percentage of non-elderly Americans covered by employment-based health insurance went from 67.1 percent down to 65.6 percent.[74] Despite this decrease in the number of employees who have insurance from their employers, the percentage of employers who have offered insurance to their employees increased from roughly 72.4 percent in 1987 to 76 percent in 2001.[75] One group that has undergone substantial loss in the area of access to health insurance is retirees, including those who have opted for early retirement. In 1993, 43 percent of early retirees were offered health insurance by large firms, while in 2001 that number dropped to 29 percent. Only 23 percent of large employers offered coverage to non-early retirees in 2001, down from 40 percent in 1993.[76] Moreover, there is evidence that lack of insurance is associated with increased risk of decline in health among retirees.[77]

Many employees are not subscribing to employer-based insurance because they cannot afford to do so, especially among small employers.[78] Employers achieved successful cost containment in health care by cost shifting to employees.[79] They guided employees into managed care plans.[80]

Many employers encouraged their employees, often through financial incentives, to opt for employee-only benefits and, in this way, to relinquish family coverage. Employees may find themselves unable to afford family coverage because employers now give only a fixed amount to each employee.[81] During the heyday of the 1980s, large corporations that paid health-care benefits tended to pay the full amount.

There are other forms of cost shifting to employees. Some employers cap their total benefits contribution, requiring employees to choose between, for example, health and pension benefits, by providing health benefits that dramatically reduced services such as prescription drugs and psychiatric benefits, and increasing the amount of deductibles and co-payments.[82] Employee contribution to 'employer-provided' health care is also high.[83] One foundation's study found that in 1996 employees paid roughly 30 percent of the total premium.[84] More recently, in 2000 and 2001, this figure hovered around 27 percent for family coverage.[85] Not surprisingly, the cost to employees has left lower-income and part-time employees unable to afford the insurance offered to them.[86] Thus, although costs were contained in the 1990s, there was widespread cost shifting to employees and the shepherding of employees into managed care which, itself, often involves significant cost-shifting practices, such as 'cherry picking' and aggressively implemented medical-necessity review. Although there is a movement to improve quality in health care, employers have reduced the rates of reimbursement to providers, in effect undermining their ability to deliver high-quality care to patients.[87]

Fueled by escalating health-care costs and the backlash against managed care, there has also been a move by employers to limit their obligation to provide health insurance through the use of what has been called 'consumer driven' health care.[88] In the most extreme version of this, employers would give their employees vouchers to purchase coverage. In other versions, employers make defined contributions to a 'personal health account' combined with catastrophic insurance. Employees are able to draw on this account to purchase health-care services with tax-exempt dollars. In the overly optimistic words of one health policy scholar, this kind of plan facilitates 'a rational health-care system that can meet the needs of each family. It is not a one-tiered, two-tiered, or even five- or six-tiered health-care system. It is a 270-million-tiered health-care system that delivers exactly those services each individual demands.'[89] An approach of this kind may enhance choice; it may also be burdensome for the sickest patients who may be less able to find plans that will spread risk within a price range that they can afford. Although this problem may be preventable through careful plan design, it is too soon to predict the success of this approach.[90]

Given what we have learned from the social experiment with managed care, it would seem that consumer-driven plans would only exacerbate already familiar problems. As we saw in Chapter 4, social relations that are more or less equal may also be health-promoting. Consumer-driven health care, though promising more choice in principle, may result in less de facto choice for consumers—as they attempt to navigate the complexities of the health-insurance marketplace within the confines of a limited budget. Many of the sickest patients will find it difficult to benefit from risk-pooling practices in consumer-driven schemes. Thus, although organizations may want to limit their obligations to their employees by embracing employee choice through consumer-driven plans, doing so may only make matters worse, both within the workplace and within the larger community. Thus, consumer-driven health insurance may not be in the best interest of subscribers.

The trend in cost shifting does not bode well for employers. Instead of acting as ethically responsible proxies, employers seem to be moving in the direction of abandoning their proxy responsibilities. This is most evident in the recent preference for consumer-driven health care. Increasingly, employers seem focused on the best interest of the organization and its shareholders, and not the beneficiaries of the care.[91] As the labor market loosened, employers moved away from giving generous health plans.[92] It is difficult to see how the direction employers have taken could constitute substituted judgment. Many employees now cannot afford the health insurance that their employers offer them.[93] Although wage growth and inflation have remained relatively stable over the last 13 years, both under 5 percent, health-plan increases in employer premiums reached 11 percent in 2001.[94] Few employees, however, would choose to have either themselves or their families without health insurance altogether. Surveys indicate that patients value a high-trust relationship with their physicians and employees value choice, continuity of care, and quality—features often not present in the managed-care plans preferred by employers. Other surveys show a distinct concern by subscribers with managed care—especially strictly managed care.[95] Moreover, the backlash against managed care and the move by employees into more flexible plans reflect their rejection of a tightly managed care system. Substituted judgment would seem to imply, among other things, that employers should not shepherd their employees into a single HMO, but instead find an array of plans with substantially different benefits from which employees can choose. Although it is too soon to know for certain, consumer-driven care may not reflect the choices patients would make despite its name.[96] If patients are not in a financial position to afford the many options offered by consumer-driven plans, such plans may be meaningless to them.

The best-interest-of-the-employee test fares no better here. At the very least, employees' interests are served by having health insurance while the trend among employers has been to price these benefits beyond the reach of many employees. If health plans are not within the financial wherewithal of employees, then their interests quite simply are not being served. Employees also need a trusting doctor–patient relationship, which is often missing in aggressively managed medicine.[97] They are best served by health insurance that fosters continuity of patient care, and a competent doctor enabled by a benefit plan to provide adequate care.[98] Care that is delivered efficiently and without undue burden, such as lengthy trips to remote facilities, is also in their interest. Finally, it is in the interest of employees to have care that respects them as persons—in the full moral sense of the term. This includes preserving patient privacy and confidentiality and respecting patients' rights to information. Although these characteristics are uncontroversially in the interest of patients, many of them are not adequately present in the health-care plans crafted by employers.

So far I have spoken of the implications of proxy criteria for substantive benefits. But another issue to which these criteria are relevant, and which I want to turn to briefly, has to do with the eligibility criteria for health benefits. Typically, only full-time employees are eligible for benefits. Thus retirees, contract, and part-time employees may be excluded from these plans. Chances are that if we apply either the best-interest-of-the-employee test or substituted judgment to the question of whether these employees should receive health benefits, the answer would be 'yes.' Given the opportunity, many currently non-eligible employees would, no doubt, express a desire to have employer-based insurance and, in this way, would qualify should the question be raised under substituted judgment. Moreover, in the absence of radical reform of the health-care system, employer-based health insurance is in the best interest of employees since they may not otherwise have insurance.

Employer decision making with respect to health benefits does not adequately reflect either substituted judgment, nor the best-interest-of-the-employee. Instead, and perhaps not surprisingly in light of the fiduciary duties of many organizations, decisions about employer-based insurance seem to reflect a narrowly construed concern with the best interest of the organization. Arguably, a decision about how to distribute health-care benefits should reflect the health and wishes of the individuals to be served. Once the decision to provide benefits has been made, it is governed by certain implicit standards.

Peele et al. looked at the role of employers as agents for employees and found employers' performance satisfactory with respect to their agency responsibilities.[99] They based their conclusion on three kinds of data: interviews with human resource managers, focus groups with employees, and a review of information distributed by employers about benefits. They evaluated employers *qua* agents on the basis of three criteria: (1) employer understanding of employee preferences, (2) incorporation of employee preferences into health plans, and (3) employees valuing their employer's role as agent in purchasing health plans. In some respects, these criteria reflect substituted judgment. The study's findings are interesting. With respect to the employee preferences, two health-plan characteristics stood out as important for 88 employees in focus groups: (1) specific providers in the plan and (2) quality of care. Significantly less important, but still identified by the

employees were: amount of employee premium and covered services.[100]
Employers identified employee preferences as follows: access to providers was
most important, then out-of-pocket costs, employee portion of premiums,
dependent's portion, perceived quality of care, and last, HMO accreditation.

Although there appears to be significant variations among employees and
employers on what employees prefer, according to Peele et al., there was
great consistency among the five employers who participated in focus
groups. Within this subset of employers, access to providers and quality of
care were both rated highly.[101] Thus, read in the best light, there is some evidence of consistency. The investigators also found that employers incorporate the preferences of employees insofar as they offer a number of different
plans, including plans with an expansive network of providers.

In view of this, Peele et al. conclude that employers are for the most part
meeting their agency responsibilities.[102] From my reading, however, they did
not assess whether employers took quality of care into account. Indeed, they
note that none of the employers provided them with the data that would
have permitted an assessment of quality (HEDIS, satisfaction survey).[103]
Given the high ratings employees gave to quality and the potential impact
plan incentives may have on physician conduct and, in turn, quality, this
seems like a significant omission. Moreover, 98 percent of employer respondents indicated that the cost of the plan was the most important factor that
they *actually* took into account in selecting plans.[104] It is difficult to see how
one could conclude that employers are meeting their agency obligations
without information about quality of care provided by the plans, especially
when the cost of the plan is such an important consideration for employers.

Employer leadership in exercising discretion

Employers may believe that since they are not bound by ERISA to provide
particular benefits, they therefore have complete discretion to decide what
benefits to provide employees. This assumption betrays confusion about the
nature of discretion. In effect, decisions about what health benefits employees have are decisions that will determine the specific care individuals
receive. Workplace rationing and bedside rationing now work together in
determining the care patients will receive. The fact that employers now participate in these decisions does not mean that they should be made at the
unfettered discretion of the employer. To draw this conclusion is to mis-
construe the notion of 'discretion.' I have suggested that the standards
employers should use when making benefits choices for their employees are
those usually used by proxies in the clinical context.

In a discussion of judicial activism, Ronald Dworkin distinguishes
between two kinds of discretion—weak and strong. According to Dworkin,
context is important for knowing what kind of discretion is at issue.
Sometimes discretion is weak, which is to say that the standards the decision-maker needs to use cannot be applied mechanically. For example, if a

decision-maker is asked to choose 'the most experienced people,' she may have discretion to construe the word 'experienced.' Decision-makers also have weak discretion when they have what amounts to the final say. An umpire's decision at a baseball game is a good example of the latter. A person can be said to have strong discretion when not bound by the standards of a particular authority, as when asked simply to choose any five people. In all three instances, however, Dworkin underscores that the decision-maker is bound by 'certain standards of rationality, fairness and effectiveness.'[105] Consider this as applied to employer-based insurance. Employers may have discretion in the strong sense when it comes to choosing health-care benefits since, given ERISA, they are virtually without any authority to prescribe substantive benefits. Nonetheless, this is not to say that there are no standards relevant to what they decide.

Employers are, after all, dealing with health care and with proxy decision making, both of which import certain ethical standards from the medical context. In addition, their actions in this sphere can affect our collective interest in social capital. When employers pay so little for benefits that health plans are unable to provide quality care in a trust-rich, doctor–patient relationship, and when they contract with health plans that employ unsavory cost containment mechanisms, then their use of discretion is not consistent with what Dworkin calls 'standards of rationality, fairness and effectiveness.' More specifically, their choices are inconsistent with the ethical standards to which proxy decision-makers are held.[106]

The argument from social capital

I have argued that employers are proxies with respect to their employees. Applied to health care this means that employers should provide a health-care plan that meets employee needs and wishes. Special attention should be paid to patient choice. Part of what drives a desire for choice is the wish of patients to choose their physician and to remain with trusted physicians.[107] But choice may be important not only because it allows patients to receive their care from a trusted physician, but also because of what it symbolizes. Giving consumers choice signals that their preferences, concerns, interests, and desires are important. Depriving them of choice may convey the opposite message—it may signal a lack of concern for them. Naturally, given what is at issue here—care, concern, and trust, the decision made by payers/employers about how many plans to offer and what kind—will itself either foster social capital or have a chilling effect on its development.

Employers who offer plans that include provisions for extensive patient choice and relative autonomy by physicians will not only improve patient satisfaction, but will also contribute to our reservoir of social capital. There is good evidence that when patients have adequate choice of physicians they are more likely to trust them. Moreover, patient trust in their health plan is positively associated with trust in their physician.[108] The findings of

Enthoven et al. also speak to this matter. They found greater consumer satisfaction in the presence of a choice of plans that include wide access plans at an equal or lower cost than the other plans offered.[109] Let us think about these findings from the perspective of trust, social relations, equality, and social capital. From the perspective of subscribers, this scenario has an equalizing aspect; it puts both kinds of plans within the financial wherewithal of most employees. In a wide-access plan, some employees will receive more health care than others, not because they have paid more, but for reasons having to do with their preferences and satisfaction.[110] This strategy creates more trust between employers and subscribers and facilitates increased trust between patients and physicians. Chances are it also increases trust among employees because there will be greater equality with respect to health care. In this way, greater choice will contribute positively to social capital levels.

An organization that meets the more demanding obligations imposed by proxy criteria may have reduced profits as a result.[111] Moreover, meeting these obligations to employees may go beyond what we have come to expect from employers. Why should an employer undertake this extra commitment? I have argued that they should undertake it because it is part of what is involved in being a proxy. I also suggest that reconsidering the purpose for which employers offer health benefits indicates that it is in their business interest to do so.[112] But there are other reasons as well. Employers owe it to themselves and to the community to enhance and maintain high levels of social capital. Providing subscribers with medical care that is rich in trust and social capital will help organizations replenish our collective and mutual fund of social capital. It will benefit not only patients and the community, but also organizations such as employers and insurers.

Organizations depend on social capital because they rely on cooperative activity in order to conduct business. Families and other close relationships draw less on trust for cooperation than do large organizations because frequent interactions carry frequent occasions to change one's views, right a past wrong or misunderstanding, or, in the worst case scenario, exact punishment. Organizations, however, are typically characterized by vertical and hierarchical relationships in which people may see each other infrequently, and trust is, in turn, more difficult to come by.[113] In place of trust, organizations can use monitoring mechanisms, such as supervisors, but they are not always reliable and can be expensive. Trust is a less expensive and more effective alternative to supervisors. Moreover, as the nature of work itself changes, moving toward a team approach, the need for trust will be greater. Thus organizations are poor producers of trust and social capital, yet relatively high users.

Trust is a valuable resource for organizations, because it is the 'superglue' that allows for cooperative activity and organizations depend upon cooperation. Trust is good for business. Organizations that are trusted will have a competitive advantage because they will benefit from improved inter-firm relations. George Brenkert points out that where there is trust among firms, they are more likely to share technology, marketing information, facilities, and employee talents.[114] Of course, customers will not do business with firms they do not trust and will take their business elsewhere. Organizations know that they need the public's trust. Brenkert identifies a number of advertising companies that speak to the efforts of organizations to secure public trust. Sears drew customers to its financial services by saying, 'Trust Sears to make it work for you,' and the American Automobile Association implores customers to 'Travel with someone you trust.'[115] And as we know from Chapter 3, some health plans piggyback on the trust that patients have for their physicians and regularly invoke it in their advertisements. Others have found that retailers that have a high level of trust in the manufacturer generate sales, up to 78 percent more.[116] There is little controversy that trust and social capital have the potential to reduce transaction costs and increase profits.[117] It is also pretty clear that organizations, and especially large vertical ones, are not significant producers of trust. Nor are they purchasing it on the open market. Kenneth Arrow nicely frames the problem with trust in the following passage.[118]

> Now trust has a very important and pragmatic value. . . . Trust is an important lubricant of a social system. It is extremely efficient; . . . unfortunately, this is not a commodity that can be bought very easily . . . trust and similar values, loyalty or truth-telling, are examples of what the economist calls 'externalities.' They are goods, they are commodities; they have real, practical, economic value; they increase the efficiency of the system, enable you to produce more goods or more of whatever values you hold in high esteem. But they are not commodities for which trade of them on the open market is technically possible or ever meaningful.

Arrow's point, that trust is a real commodity, but one which cannot be bought and sold, has important normative implications. Although it cannot be bought and sold, it can be stolen. That is, it can be taken without fair exchange. As I described in Chapter 3, trust is a social good, subject to the free-rider problem. The community, including its families, professional relationships, schools, and civic and voluntary associations, produces relatively high levels of trust through its various activities. Organizations, in general low producers of trust, nonetheless draw on the trust that is available in the community. In the case of aggressively managed health plans, however, the situation is bleak since at the same time that MCOs use trust to lubricate the organization, they undermine an important source of trust and social capital, namely the doctor–patient relationship. It is worth keeping in mind that managed care has been a relatively profitable business. For example, the CEOs of HMOs anticipate making about 62 percent more than the CEOs of other similarly sized corporations.[119]

State legislation that targets some of the problems associated with employer-based health insurance offers little hope of change. State mandates, such as freedom-of-choice laws, mandatory inclusion provisions, mandatory minimums for hospital stays, and mandatory coverage for certain groups, will not reach the many Americans already in ERISA-governed, self-insured plans. Moreover, when expensive mandates are enacted in the shadow of ERISA they may drive employers to self-insure and, in this way, avoid the reach of state insurance law.[120] Thus, state mandates are not likely to result in substantially improved benefits for subscribers.

This problem is exacerbated by the fact that ERISA's preemption includes within its net the mechanism that typically functions to monitor medicine—namely, malpractice litigation, at least with respect to mixed medical benefits cases. Nonetheless, legislation, such as that enacted by Texas in 1997, which would permit patients to sue their MCOs, may provide some relief to potential litigants.[121] Many other states have introduced similar legislation.[122] But it is not yet clear whether these laws will be preempted by ERISA. Federal mandates, including the recently enacted Mental Health Parity Act (1996) and the Newborn and Mothers Health Protection Act (1996), supersede ERISA and thus apply to self-insured plans.[123] These may signal increased and much needed federal involvement in health care.

At present, traditional economic theory understands employers' benefits, including health-care benefits, as a form of compensation. And, indeed, historically, health care was given to employees instead of pay raises, at a time when pay raises were frozen. These benefits have become so firmly entrenched that they are now viewed by many more as a right than as a privilege.[124] Thus, if employers price benefits so high that employees can no longer afford to take them, then employees are losing that compensation and employers are, in turn, receiving that portion of their labor free of charge. Although perhaps unintended, the consequence of this is to treat employee labor as slave labor representing the worst kind of exploitation. I have argued that although ERISA, rightly or wrongly, puts the question of what substantive benefits belong in employee-benefits packages in the hands of employers, it does not follow that employers have unfettered discretion.

I have argued in support of the view that employers are under an obligation to assume increased moral responsibility for the substance of health benefits and, in particular, a rich doctor–patient relationship. First, I argued that in their capacity as proxy decision-makers for their employees, both substituted judgment and best interest speak for this enhanced obligation. In particular, there is evidence both that employees would choose a trust-rich doctor–patient relationship and that such a relationship is in their best interest. Second, fairness considerations mandate that employers contribute a fair share to our collective reservoir of social capital. Third, in view of the considerable benefits to be had from increased social capital, there are consequentialist reasons in support of this specific obligation.

Ultimately, we cannot treat health care just like any other commodity;

we cannot sever it from the meaning it has acquired in our community. Nor would it be desirable to do so. Of course, providing a trust-rich doctor–patient relationship will come at a cost to the organizations that must pay for it, most of which are driven by the need to produce profits for shareholders. The question to be asked is why the burden of producing social capital should rest on the shoulders of these organizations. Arguably, since facilitating social capital would appear to carry some burdens with it, those burdens should be distributed fairly across industries. To some extent, a broad distribution of this burden occurs when employers/payers assume the greater financial responsibility associated with meeting their proxy obligations. Nonetheless, health plans may assume an even greater role than payers.

Trust and social capital create a number of benefits, such as the increased capacity for cooperative activity, that benefit both individuals and organizations. But trust and social capital also improve health outcomes. If the vast public health literature speaking to this is right, then we would anticipate a healthier population and, in turn, lower health-care costs because of increased social capital. In other words, we may select health plans among other organizations, for the special responsibility of creating social capital, because they are uniquely situated to benefit from our reservoir of social capital.

However, health plans are also well situated to produce social capital. They work through physicians and other healing professionals—people in whom community members have historically invested trust. Medicine has historically symbolized many of the values associated with social capital, including concern for others, healing, and caring. Because of this, health plans are strategically positioned to either exploit that vessel of trust for private gain or conserve it as a public resource. They have the wherewithal to either destroy the doctor–patient relationship as a source of social capital, or contribute to its capacity to create this public good. Finally, a society committed to improving public policy through close attention to social capital will reflect on the ability of institutions to create and maintain social capital.

Notes

1 J. Gabel et al. Job-based Benefits in 2002: Some Important Trends. *Health Affairs*, 2002; 21: 143.
2 *The Employment Retirement Income Security Act*, 88 Stat. 832, P.L. 93–406, 29 U.S.C. 1001 et seq. (2005).
3 H.M. Sapolsky et al. Corporate Attitudes Toward Health Care Costs. *Milbank Memorial Fund Quarterly*, 1981; 59: 570.
4 H.M. Sapolsky. Empire and the Business of Health Insurance. *Journal of Health Politics, Policy and Law*, 1991; 16: 749.
5 R. Kronick and T. Gilmer. Explaining the Decline in Health Insurance Coverage, 1979–1995. *Health Affairs*, 1999; 18: 45.

6 I do not take up the interesting question of whether employers would be bound by standards were benefits mere gifts. Arguably, though, such a case could be made.

7 T.A. Brennan. An Ethical Perspective on Health Care Insurance Reform. *American Journal of Law and Medicine*, 1993; 19: 48.

8 Ibid., p. 51.

9 Ibid.

10 Ibid., p. 52.

11 Ibid.

12 M. Angell and J. Kassirer. Quality and the Medical Marketplace—Following Elephants. *New England Journal of Medicine*, 1996; 335: 883–5.

13 R. Kuttner. The American Health Care System: Employee-Sponsored Health Coverage. *New England Journal of Medicine*, 1999; 340: 251.

14 *Black's Law Dictionary*, 6th edn. St. Paul: West Publishing Co., 1990, p. 1226.

15 *Cruzan v. Director Missouri Department of Health*, 497 U.S. 261, 1990.

16 Because larger firms tend to offer more than one plan, and most employees work in larger firms, 60 percent of covered employees can choose among plans. Still many of those working in small and medium-size firms have little choice. Kaiser Family Foundation. *Chartbook: Trends and Indicators in the Changing Health Care Marketplace*, May 2002, p. 19.

17 T. Bodenheimer and K. Sullivan. How Large Employers are Shaping the Health Care Marketplace. *New England Journal of Medicine*, 1998; 338: 1004.

18 M. Suszynski, Health Insurers Face the Heat. *Best's Review*, March 2003, p. 12; M. Green, Managed Choice. *Best's Review*, MA: 2003, pp. 71–6.

19 Gabel et al., op. cit., pp. 143–51.

20 Kaiser Family Foundation and Health Research and Educational Trust. *Employer Health Benefits 2004 Annual Survey*, September 2004, Chart #7.

21 Kaiser Family Foundation and Health Research and Educational Trust, ibid., Chart #1.

22 Ibid.

23 Gabel et al., op. cit., pp. 143–51.

24 Kaiser Family Foundation and Health Research and Educational Trust, op. cit., Chart #5.

25 Gabel et al., op. cit., pp. 143–51.

26 Ibid.

27 CNN.com. *G.E. Workers Strike Over Health Care Costs*, XIV January 2003, online, available at: <http://www.cnn.com> (accessed 2003).

28 Kaiser Family Foundation and Health Research and Educational Trust, op. cit., Chart #1.

29 Ibid.

30 S. Heffler et al. Health Spending Projections Through 2013. *Health Affairs*, 11 February 2004, Web Exclusive W4, pp. 79–93.

31 J.B. Christianson. The Role of Employers In Community Healthcare Systems. *Health Affairs*, 1998; 7: 163.

32 See, for example, E.H. Morreim. *Balancing Act: The New Medical Ethics of Medicine's New Economics*. Washington, DC: Georgetown University Press, 1995.

33 Bodenheimer and Sullivan, op. cit., p. 1005.

34 Ibid.

35 L.D. Schaeffer and L.C. Volpe. Focusing on the Health Care Consumer. *Health Affairs*, 1999; 18: 27.

36 J.C. Robinson. The Future of Managed Care Organization. *Health Affairs*, 1999; 18: 10.

37 Ibid.
38 *The Employment Retirement Income Security Act of 1974*, 88 Stat. 832 P.L. 93–406, 29 U.S.C. 1001 et seq. (2005).
39 Sapolsky, op. cit., pp. 747–61.
40 A.A. Gawande et al. Does Dissatisfaction With Health Plans Stem From Having No Choices? *Health Affairs*, 1998; 17: 187.
41 Ibid.
42 Ibid., p. 190.
43 Ibid., p. 188.
44 P. Starr. *The Transformation of American Medicine*. New York: Basic Books, Inc., 1949, pp. 310–26.
45 Bureau of Labor Statistics. *Union Members Summary*. United States Department of Labor, Washington, DC, 25 February 2003, online, available at: <http://www.bls.gov/news.release/union2.nr0.htm> (accessed 2003).
46 D. Rosner and G. Markovitz. The Struggle over Employee Benefits: The Role of Labor in Influencing Modern Health Policy. *Milbank Quarterly*, 2003; 81: 45–68.
47 Ibid.
48 C. Montagne. Bargaining Health Benefits in the Workplace: An Inside View. *Milbank Quarterly*, 2002; 80: 547–67.
49 J. Gabel et al. Trends in Out-of-Pocket Spending by Insured American Workers 1990–1997. *Health Affairs*, 2001; 20: 47–56. See also J. Gabel et al. Job-Based Health Insurance in 2000: Premiums Rise Sharply While Coverage Grows. *Health Affairs*, 2000; 19: 144–51; Rosner and Markovitz, op. cit.
50 B.R. Furrow et al. *Health Law: Cases, Materials and Problems*. St Paul: West Publishing Co., 1997, pp. 1105–13.
51 Ibid.
52 Ibid.
53 Gawande et al., op. cit., p. 190.
54 K. Donelan et al. The Cost of Health System Change: Public Discontent in Five Nations. *Health Affairs*, 1999; 18: p. 209.
55 Ibid., p. 213.
56 Gawande et al., op. cit., p. 190.
57 Ibid.
58 A. Enthoven et al. Consumer Choice and the Managed Care Backlash. *American Journal of Law and Medicine*, 2001; 27: 6.
59 Kaiser Family Foundation/Harvard School of Public Health. National Survey of Consumer Experiences with and Attitudes Toward Health Plans, August 2001.
60 K. Grumbach et al. Resolving the Gatekeeper Conundrum: What Patients Value in Primary Care and Referrals to Specialists. *Journal of the American Medical Association*, 1999; 282: 261–6.
61 M. Freudenheim. HMOs Cope with a Backlash on Cost Cutting. *New York Times*, 19 May 1996, Sec. 1; T. Bodenheimer. The HMO Backlash—Righteous or Reactionary? *New England Journal of Medicine*, 1996; 335: 1602.
62 Ibid.
63 R. Blendon et al. Understanding the Managed Care Backlash. *Health Affairs*, 1998; 17: 84.
64 Kaiser/Harvard PSRA Poll (22 August 1997), as described in Blendon et al., op. cit., pp. 80–110.
65 M. Hall et al. How Disclosing HMO Physician Incentives Affects Trust. *Health Affairs*, 2002; 21: 197–206.
66 V. Tweed. Making HMOs Compete. *Business Health*, 1994; 12: 27–38.
67 E. O'Brien. Employers' Benefits from Workers' Health Insurance. *Milbank Quarterly*, 2003; 81: 5.
68 Ibid., p. 11.
69 Ibid., p. 24.

70 Ibid., pp. 5–43.
71 Hall et al. op. cit.
72 Kronick and Gilmer, op. cit., p. 31; Kuttner, op. cit., p. 248.
73 P. Fronstin. *Employment-Based Health Benefits: Trends and Outlook*. EBRI Issue Brief #233, May 2001, p. 3. Online, available at: <http://www.ebri.com> (accessed 2003).
74 P. Fronstin. *Sources of Health Insurance*. EBRI Issue Brief # 252, December 2002. Online, available at: <http://www.ebri.com> (accessed 2003).
75 P.F. Cooper and B.S. Schone. More Offers, Fewer Takers for Employment Based Health Insurance 1987–1997. *Health Affairs*, 1997; 16: 144; Fronstin, op. cit.
76 J.K. Iglehart. Changing Health Insurance Trends. *New England Journal of Medicine*, 2002; 347: 956–62.
77 D.W. Baker et al. Lack of Health Insurance and Decline in Overall Health in Late Middle Age. *New England Journal of Medicine*, 2001; 345: 1106–12.
78 P. Fronstin et al. *Small Employers and Health Benefits: Findings from the 2002 Small Employer Health Benefits Survey*. EBRI Issue Brief # 253, January 2003. Online, available at: <http://www.ebri.com> (accessed 2003).
79 Kuttner, op. cit., p. 248; Iglehart, op. cit.
80 Kuttner, op. cit., p. 249.
81 Ibid.
82 Ibid.
83 Ibid.
84 E. O'Brien and J. Feder. Employment-Based Coverage and its Decline: The Growing Plight of Low-Wage Workers. Prepared for the Kaiser Commission on Medicaid and the Uninsured, Washington, DC: Henry J. Kaiser Foundation, May 1999.
85 Kaiser Family Foundation, op. cit., p. 30.
86 General Accounting Office. *Employment-Based Health Insurance: Costs Increase and Family Coverage Decreases* (GAO/ HEHS-97–35). Washington, DC: Government Printing Office, February 1997, p. 2.
87 T. Bodenheimer. The Movement for Improved Quality in Health Care. *New England Journal of Medicine*, 1999; 340: 492.
88 Iglehart, op. cit.
89 See J. Robinson. The End of Managed Care. *Journal of the American Medical Association*, 2001; 285: 2623.
90 T.W. Samuel et al. The Next Stage in the Health Care Economy: Aligning the Interests of Patients, Providers, and Third-Party Payers Through Consumer-Driven Health Plans. *American Journal of Surgery*, 2003; 186: 117–24.
91 MCOs report that price is more important than patient satisfaction or quality of care in successful negotiation with employers. R. Bergman. Study: Employers Consider Cost Over Quality in Health Purchases. *Hospitals and Health Networks*, 1994; 68: 54.
92 Iglehart, op. cit.
93 K.E. Thorpe et al. Why Are Workers Uninsured? Employer-Sponsored Health Insurance in 1997. *Health Affairs*, 1999; 18: 213–18.
94 Kaiser Family Foundation, op. cit., p. 28.
95 Kaiser Family Foundation/Harvard School of Public Health, op. cit.
96 P.B. Peele et al. Employer-Sponsored Health Insurance: Are Employers Good Agents for Their Employees? *Milbank Quarterly*, 2000; 78: pp. 5–21.
97 B. Gray. Trust and Trustworthy Care in the Managed Care Era. *Health Affairs*, 1997; 16: 35.
98 E.J. Emanuel and N. Neveloff Dubler. Preserving the Physician–Patient Relationship in the Era of Managed Care. In *Contemporary Issues in Bioethics*,

5th edn ed. T.L. Beauchamp and L. Walters. Belmont, CA: Wadsworth Publishing Company, 1999, pp. 389–99.

99 Peele et al., op. cit.
100 Ibid., p. 12.
101 Ibid., pp. 13–14.
102 Ibid., p. 19.
103 Ibid., p. 15.
104 Ibid., p. 17.
105 R. Dworkin. The Model of Rules. In *Taking Rights Seriously*. Cambridge, MA: Harvard University Press, 1978, p. 31.
106 For a discussion of how employers can both meet enhanced duties to employees while at the same time meeting their fiduciary obligations to stockholders, see P. Illingworth. A Role for Stakeholder Ethics in Meeting the Ethical Challenges Posed by Managed-Care Organizations. *HEC Forum*, 1999; 11: 306–22.
107 Bodenheimer and Sullivan, op. cit., p. 1007.
108 A.C. Kao et al. The Relationship Between Method of Physician Payment and Patient Trust. *Journal of the American Medical Association*, 1998; 280: 1708–14.
109 Enthoven et al., op. cit.
110 At the same time, one needs to be careful not to take away with one hand what one has given with the other. Policy-makers need to keep in mind that inequalities in health care may diminish social capital and the benefits to be had from equal social relations.
111 Clearly, if O'Brien is right and providing health benefits is in the business interest of an organization, this is not necessarily the case. E. O'Brien. Employers' Benefits from Workers' Health Insurance. *Milbank Quarterly*, 2003; 81: 5–43.
112 Ibid.
113 R. La Porta et al. Trust in Large Organizations. *AEA Papers and Proceedings*, 1997; 87: 333–8; R. Putnam. *Making Democracy Work: Civic Tradition in Modern Italy*. Princeton: Princeton University Press, 1993.
114 G. Brenkert. Marketing Trust: Barriers and Bridges. *Business and Professional Ethics Journal*, 1997; 16: 78.
115 Ibid., p. 79.
116 N. Kumar. The Power of Trust in Manufacturer–Retailer Relationships. *Harvard Business Review*, 1996; 97: 92–106.
117 F. Fukuyama. *Trust: The Social Virtues and the Creation of Prosperity*. New York: The Free Press, 1995, p. 26.
118 K. Arrow. Uncertainty and the Welfare Economics of Medical Care. *The American Economic Review*, 1963; LIII: 851–83.
119 Bodenheimer. The HMO Backlash—Righteous or Reactionary?, op. cit.
120 G.A. Jenson and M.A. Morrisey. Employer Sponsored Health Insurance and Mandated Benefit Laws. *Milbank Quarterly*, 1999; 77: 441.
121 Texas Civ. Prac. & Rem. Code § 88.002 (1999).
122 M. Stauffer and Donald R. Levy (eds). *State by State Guide to Managed Care Law*. New York: Aspen Publishers Inc., 2000, pp. 5.49–5.65.
123 The other federal mandates that supercede ERISA are the: Pregnancy Discrimination Act (1978), Consolidated Omnibus Budget Reconciliation Act (1985 COBRA), Health Insurance Portability and Accountability Act (HIPAA), 1996.
124 L.D. Schaeffer and L.C. Volpe. Focusing on the Health Care Consumers. *Health Affairs*, 1999; 18: 26.

8 Protecting medical trust, conserving social capital

As of 2004, both the cost of health care and the cost of health insurance continue to rise.[1] In 2003, 45 million Americans did not have health insurance.[2] With costs on the rise and in the midst of a recession, employers/payers are considering a change in the nature of their involvement in the nation's health care. Yet, there is no sign of a move toward a national health insurance program. Though enrollment in managed care had declined, it seems again to be stabilizing. Nonetheless, there appears to be increased interest by employers in consumer-driven plans.[3] Indeed, the recently enacted Medicare Prescription Drug Improvement and Modernization Act of 2003 included the creation of legislation providing for tax-deductible health savings accounts.[4] No one knows whether federal protection of managed care will continue. Although the Supreme Court in *Kentucky Association of Health Plans v. Miller* surprised many with its protection of any-willing-provider laws and, in turn, the relationship between doctor and patient,[5] its decision in *Aetna Health, Inc. v. Davila*[6] does not bode well for the doctor–patient relationship.

As we continue to think about health policy and the values that underlie it, there are some lessons to be learned from the analysis of this book. Trust conservation is important not only for the doctor–patient relationship, but also for the cultivation of social capital. In this respect, the doctor–patient relationship should be looked upon as a public good. Once social capital is taken into account, cost containment mechanisms that impair trust between doctor and patient may turn out not to be cost effective. Moreover, including social capital in the evaluation of health policy in general, and reimbursement strategies in particular, changes the nature of the moral dialog from one with a focus on the duties of private contractors to one with a focus on the welfare of the community.

In this last chapter, I will review both the cost benefit and fairness arguments in favor of a trust-rich, doctor–patient relationship. Then I will suggest some strategies for rebuilding trust. Following this, I will argue for complete transparency with respect to financial incentives, despite the threat to trust posed by such transparency. Finally, I will consider some alternative approaches to cost-effective care that have been used by employers and that appear not to compromise trust between doctor and patient.

Health plans and employers are under a moral imperative to be mindful of the consequences of their decisions for social capital, especially when these burden the relationship between patient and physician. This obligation is supported by prudential and fairness considerations. A community rich in social capital is more likely to be a healthier one and, in turn, may be one in which health care is less expensive.[7] A number of parties will benefit from this. Employers, with an interest in promoting the interests of their employees and the community, may be better able to do both in the context of a trust-rich environment. Continuing to shift the cost of health benefits to employees, especially when they may have to refuse the benefit or strike, as 19,000 General Electric employees did in the post-9/11 months, would seem not to be in anyone's interest.[8] Such strikes are likely to decrease trust and social capital not only between employer and employee, but also between employers and the communities in which they reside.

Employers have a choice about whether or not to provide benefits that permit a trust-rich doctor–patient relationship and, in turn, social capital. In Chapter 7, I argued that they should be guided by proxy duties in their role as plan designers. There are also prudential and fairness reasons for thinking that they should be mindful of social capital. Employers are high users of trust and social capital. They use social capital within their organizations, between the organization and other organizations, and with the community. Yet, as we saw, large organizations are not significant producers of trust and social capital. They may use more than their fair share (more than they have contributed). If this is so and in fact they are profiting from the fact that others are behaving in ways that are conducive to the production of trust and social capital, then employers may have a moral duty to act in ways that will increase their contribution of social capital. Otherwise they risk free riding on the contribution of others to the social capital fund. Health-plan design offers employers an opportunity to reciprocate.

Health plans may also benefit from using cost containment strategies that protect trust. As I discussed in Chapter 5, there is evidence that social-capital-rich communities confer benefits on health plans that increase the likelihood that patients in managed plans are better able to tolerate compromised trust between doctor and patient.[9] If so, then it would seem to follow that managed plans have a direct and financial interest in conducting business in a way that will contribute to social capital levels. A safe prediction is that when a sub-study is undertaken it will show that social-capital-rich communities also confer greater trust on employers/payers. To some extent, this follows conceptually from the fact that trust is a non-excludable public good. Still, it would be interesting to see some empirical work on this.

Employers may focus narrowly on the bottom line because of the utility of focusing on shareholder benefit. But the arguments from social capital suggest that employers and health plans should adjust their cost-benefit calculations to incorporate the additional externalities (costs) associated with their low-trust health plans. It would not be surprising if overall producing high levels of social capital were in the interest of employers. Increased social capital would have the potential to improve employer relations with and among employees, between organizations, and between organizations and their markets. It is shortsighted of employers and plans to ignore the many ways that they can generate the social capital on which they themselves depend and from which they benefit. In this book, I also argued that health plans may have a special duty to increase social capital because social capital has direct benefits with respect to health. People who have plenty of social capital tend to have better health outcomes. Therefore health plans can *uniquely* benefit from increases in trust and social capital.

Building trust and social capital by way of health-care benefits is also likely to maximize utility. Although the short-term costs of trust-rich medicine may appear to be high, in the long run the costs of health care may be less. High-trust doctor–patient relationships may be less expensive in part because they will contribute to improving health outcomes indirectly by way of the trust and social capital that they create. Not only will patients receive the therapeutic benefits of the relationship, but they are likely to be more compliant with doctors' orders and be less likely to seek outside second opinions, repeat readings of tests, etc.—all of which are costly. Moreover, they will enjoy the many benefits, including health benefits, from enriched social capital.

Despite the many benefits to accrue to health plans and employers from a trust-rich doctor–patient relationship, a 'carrot and stick' approach may be required to increase the adoption of a trust-rich approach to health care. To begin with, the benefits to the community from trust-rich plans should be acknowledged. Just as consumers reward environmentally-friendly companies with their business, so they may decide to reward social-capital-friendly organizations. Unless, however, they are aware of the considerable community benefits from trust, they will be in no position to lobby for their interests.

The public needs to be educated about social capital. A public health campaign should be undertaken celebrating the benefits of trust and social capital. Consumers should be taught how to evaluate providers and organizations on the basis of their ability to cultivate social capital. Obviously, plans that use incentives that result in alienating plan members from family and social support systems, such as those discussed in Chapter 4 in connection with the baby diagnosed with leukemia, should be discouraged. Fragmenting family members from each other and from their communities in order to access benefits both wastes social capital and fails to cultivate additional social capital. Poorly-endowed capitated plans, which inadvertently encourage physicians to cherry pick and to reduce the time they spend with patients, may also compromise trust and social capital. To the extent that any of those incentives are unequally distributed, they may further compromise health, trust, and social capital.

It is not difficult to imagine that quality assurance programs could rate health plans for trust just as they now rate them for safety. Since trust is an increasingly measurable phenomenon, subscribers could, given the information, evaluate their physicians and plans for their trustworthiness.[10] For this to be a worthwhile enterprise, however, patients need to understand the importance of trust and social capital for themselves, the community, and future generations. Public health campaigns that depict 'life without trust' might go a long way in conveying the importance of what is at issue. Businesses may themselves decide to celebrate their 'sensitivity to social capital' in their marketing campaigns. When campaigns invest in employee and community health through trust-rich health plans, they should advertise these plans as exemplifying good corporate citizenship. Imagine Boeing marketing their planes in the following campaign: 'Boeing: We build safe planes and safe communities with trust-rich health plans for our team members.'

In many ways, health plans that undermine trust from the doctor–patient relationship can be viewed as 'polluting' two key social resources, 'trust' and 'social capital.' The deeper the erosion of trust caused by the health plan and the more vulnerable the social capital, the stronger the case for the duty to 'restore' social capital and 'clean up' distrust. We might use a model similar to what has been used with efforts to control air pollution, such as the creative banking and trading of emissions offsets. We can imagine that, once a social capital baseline has been established, we would be better able to determine the levels of 'distrust' that different communities will be able to tolerate. Businesses that threaten social capital may be required to register with 'emissions' offices and make the case that they are implementing 'best social capital practices' in their organizations. Although such practices may strike some as mere fancy, appreciation of the profound importance of social capital for community well-being, combined with the growing ability to quantify it, may result in efforts to regulate those businesses that harm social capital through their activities.

The U.S. Department of Justice Community Policing Program constitutes another approach to restoring trust. Recognizing widespread distrust of police, the Department of Justice sought to remedy this problem by creating a partnership between the police and the community. At the heart of this program is a more visible role for neighborhood police.[11] Health plans that have used trust-compromising strategies, especially in social capital impoverished communities, may need to not only change their cost containment strategies, but also take positive steps to rebuild trust. Compensating physicians on a special fee-for-service basis to increase their time with patients and the community, for the purpose of building trust, would be a step in that direction.

Once we recognize the value of trust and social capital as social goods, and identify important sources for their cultivation, we will be better able to minimize activities that threaten trust. Having identified these industries, we can also identify 'best and worst practices' with respect to trust development.

As our ability to both measure social capital and identify specific sources improves, we will be better positioned to both build trust and to hold organizations that continue to diminish it responsible.

At this point, however, we need to recognize the importance of the doctor–patient relationship in building trust and social capital. As bioethics and other health-related disciplines come to recognize the role of social determinants in health there is a temptation to downplay the relevance of the medical arts.[12] I have argued, however, that the doctor–patient relationship and other significant healing relationships are important social determinants of health. Therefore it would be counter-productive to undermine the richness of these relationships in the name of the public's health.

But is trust between doctor and patient so important that we ought to sacrifice other goods for its sake? Indeed, the importance I have attributed to both could be marshaled in support of the conclusion that we ought to sacrifice patient self-determination for the sake of a high-trust doctor–patient relationship. To this end, some have suggested that information about trust-compromising cost containment mechanisms that might lead patients to distrust their physicians be disclosed by someone other than the physician. Health plans have been suggested.[13] The obvious problem with this suggestion is that, given the likelihood that patients will believe that their physicians will advocate for them, many patients may not understand the personal implications of the information if it is not disclosed by the physician. In the end, patient self-determination may be compromised for the sake of trust.

There are a number of other problems with this proposal. First, the proposal may fail for feasibility. Attempts to obscure relevant information might succeed only in raising suspicion and distrust about what exactly is occurring within health plans. The risk of obscuring information is that one will only succeed in conveying misinformation. Moreover, in the present context, with media attention focused on health care and the high level of knowledge that many patients have about health care, it would be difficult to ration care discreetly.

Patients cannot be counted on to refrain from asking questions, especially not in an environment in which we want to encourage them to speak openly and honestly. If they do ask questions, physicians have the choice of lying, answering vaguely, or sidestepping the question in some way. Lying to patients is unproductive in the current medical climate in which providers and administrators are committed to encouraging greater transparency.[14] Today physicians are encouraged to be open and honest with patients about, for example, medical errors and near misses. Such openness is thought to be not only a right of patients, but also the appropriate way to handle medical mistakes if one wants to reduce the harms associated with mistakes and minimize malpractice.[15] Moreover, as I argued in Chapter 2, it is unethical to lie to patients in the name of patient safety.

Given this laudable goal, it is difficult to imagine how, on the one hand, we could encourage physicians to be forthright with patients in the name of transparency yet, on the other hand, caution them not to inform patients about financial incentives. Surely the arguments that speak for transparency in the one case speak for it in the other. Presently, transparency is a priority because it is viewed as absolutely essential for identifying the causes of medical mistakes and, in turn, reducing their frequency. We could not reasonably expect to identify medical errors by way of transparency if we exclude an entire area, such as reimbursement systems, from the demands of transparency. Information about cost containment strategies, including their effect on physician behavior, is important for evaluating the success of health strategies. Such information must be part of the public domain.

Patients cannot be self-determining without information about incentives because such incentives play an important part in treatment decisions. If we review the reasons why self-determination is important for people in general and patients in particular, it can be seen that we must tell patients about rationing. According to J.S. Mill, people should be permitted to make decisions about their own case because they are in the best position to serve their own interest. They know their interests better than anyone else and are better able to position themselves to act on them.[16] This argument seems especially relevant to the very personal kinds of decisions that *patients* must make.

Although those who advocate silent rationing do so at least partially for the benefit of patients, insofar as they believe that patients will benefit from the increased trust permitted by silent rationing, it is not clear that such an approach is in the interest of patients. In the context under discussion, physicians have divided and conflicting duties. That is, they have duties to their specific patients and to a health plan and its members. Many cost containment mechanisms are also arranged so that physician reimbursement hinges on the ability of physicians to deliver care in a cost-conscious manner. Under these conditions patients may need to be their own advocates and a small dose of skepticism about their providers, plans, and care may go a long way in protecting them. This situation is very different from the traditional one in which physicians acted as fiduciaries with respect to their patients. In some plans, physicians have divided loyalties. In the face of strong conflicting interests, they cannot be counted on to be self-monitoring. In this context, patients must be more actively involved in protecting and monitoring their own care.

Patients can be more effective as monitors of their care if they have adequate information about the context, including information about the prevailing financial incentives. Without that information they may not look out for their own interests; they may not be vigilant when instructed to wait and see or seek a second opinion when the first seems amiss. Well-informed patients are in an ideal position to monitor their own well-being and medical care. And although silent rationing may maintain trust in the short term, in the end I am pessimistic that trust could flourish in such an environment. It should be underscored that trust is not incompatible with the full disclosure of *all* financial incentives; there is a tension between trust and the disclosure of specific incentives—namely, those that fall within the scope of trust based on encapsulated interest. For the most part, this will include aggressively-implemented incentives that target physician conduct. An obvious alternative to manipulating information that patients receive is to use only those economic incentives that can be used with complete transparency.

It may seem as if I am advocating that the burden of high health-care costs be borne exclusively by payers and plans. Payers could adopt inexpensive measures that might change how patients use care and at the same time preserve trust. One such approach focuses on patient self-care. Conestogo Wood Specialties, for example, responded to escalating health-care costs not only by raising their employee's co-payments, as many other employers did, but also by educating employees about when and where to seek medical care. At Conestogo, employees were educated about when to wait for a physician's office to open and when to rush to the more expensive alternative of an emergency room. This strategy has been used elsewhere and apparently with some success. After one year of implementing a program of patient education at Berk-tek, the company lowered its health-care costs by 24.3 percent per employee. Office visits dropped 18.4 percent and ER visits 19.8 percent. Much of this decrease in costs was attributed to the patient education program.[17]

At its best, a program of patient self-care carries the message of choice one step further by giving patients more control over when they go to the physician. At its worst, it encourages patients to make decisions with respect to matters over which they may have little competency. Still sometimes a cold is just a cold! Patients who are able to recognize a cold for what it is will not go running off to the doctor. An approach that targets the demand side of health care in a way that is respectful of patients, as education certainly is, is also more likely to nurture trust than one that tries to control costs by targeting the supply side, as many cost containment mechanisms do. Patient education may leave patients more empowered and, in turn, more able to trust. Empowered patients may be better able to extend trust because they feel less vulnerable. It would seem to follow that the encapsulated interest account of trust then, knowing that it is in the interest of the trustee to be trustworthy, removes some of the pressure from the entruster to self-protect. Patients who are more knowledgeable about their physicians and their health care will be in a better position both to trust their physicians and, if necessary, to withhold that trust and exercise self-trust.

Other nations may be further along in creating health-care plans that have the potential to contribute to trust and social capital. Certainly, the inclusiveness of universal health-care schemes, such as those of Canada and Britain, would seem to encourage trust and reciprocity in a way that leaving 45 million Americans without health insurance[18]—that is, uncared for—does not. Recall the discussion from Chapter 4 in which we under-scored the importance of cohesiveness and social relations for health: Durkheim, for example, stressed the importance of 'mutual moral support' in the place of 'throwing the individual on his own resources' for social cohesiveness. Nations that provide universal health care have the potential to provide the moral support that is at the heart of social cohesiveness. When the British National Health Service was enacted in 1948, it articu-lated three principles to guide the system: (1) equal access to medical care, (2) availability of comprehensive preventive and curative care, and (3) pro-vision of the service at no cost, at the point of service.[19] Together these prin-ciples have the capacity to create a climate in which people will be cared for without the feeling that their care is contingent upon their ability to pay. From the perspective of the encapsulated interest account of trust, if care will be forthcoming regardless of a patient's ability to pay, one reason for a patient to be concerned about a physician's interests is thus removed. Moreover, the principle of equal access to medical care can potentially mit-igate some of the negative impact on health associated with social status.

In Chapter 6 we spoke about the Canadian Health Act, and there explained that it emphasized the commitment of all Canadians to other Canadians. Both Canada and Great Britain are committed in principle to provide care to all their citizens, and this commitment bodes well for the cultivation of social capital. However, if the in-principle commitment is not bolstered with the funding that is actually needed to care for patients, it is little more than mere words.

Comparative studies have been done in which citizen responses to their health-care systems are surveyed. In one such survey of five nations, includ-ing Australia, Canada, New Zealand, the United Kingdom, and the United States, Blendon et al. found that those surveyed in the U.S. were signifi-cantly more likely than those surveyed in the other four countries to report problems accessing health care because of the cost of the care.[20] This is not to say that other countries do not also have access problems of one kind or another. For example, long waits for elective surgery have been reported as a major problem in the United Kingdom.[21]

Canada has similar problems. Among other problems, Canadians face a shortage of family physicians, which in turn creates long waits at clinics.[22] At the time of writing, Canada was in the midst of a health summit, addressing some of the issues raised by the Romanow Report and involving federal and provincial governments. Under negotiation was the proposal by Paul Martin, Canada's Prime Minister, to contribute funding to the provinces in exchange for (1) reduced waiting times, (2) catastrophic drug coverage, and (3) the creation of post-acute home care programs. In other words, Canada, like Britain and other countries, is struggling to improve its health-care system by infusing it with the money it needs to implement the principles it supports.[23] After several days of negotiations Martin promised the premiers and territories 18 billion dollars over 6 years for Medicare reform.[24]

The NHS's effort to reform its system reflects at least in part a recognition of the importance of the doctor–patient relationship. Following widespread dissatisfaction with the system, which had been underfunded for some time, efforts at reform were undertaken. As with Canada, perhaps the single most important step that the government took was giving the system more extensive funding.[25] The government is also committed to increasing the number of providers who will provide care for patients. The number of physicians is to be increased by 55 percent through a combination of policies, such as increasing the number of medical students and offering pay incentives and flexibility to physicians, among others.

Efforts are also being made to improve the experience of patients, such as reducing delays and giving patients a choice of physicians.[26] Recent reforms have included the establishment of national standards and targets. Some of these mandate the reduction of specific diseases, such as cancer and heart disease.[27] Others, however, target more specifically the doctor–patient relationship. For example, the government aims to cut the waiting time for NHS-funded surgery to 12 weeks by 2008 and to guarantee access to primary care physicians within two working days.[28] Measures of this kind directly target the quality of patients' experiences with their physicians, providing some of the policy support that is needed to build trust between doctor and patient and, in turn, social capital. Such a focus is likely to nurture the very ingredients necessary for patient trust, by, for example, giving physicians and patients more time together. From the point of view of cultivation of social capital, efforts of this kind should be lauded.

In this book, I have focused on 'band-aid' measures that might be applied to the current health-care system. Ultimately, however, a private health insurance system based on profit may be at odds with high levels of trust and social capital. Profit-based health insurance entails that some people are denied potentially beneficial care, so that others receive high compensation, stock options, and shareholder dividends. Differentials in treatment are especially visible in aggressively managed plans. A moral concern with this tradeoff is at the heart of the distinction between an open health-care system and a closed one.[29] In an open system, some people sacrifice beneficial care not so that others may receive care, or so that resources are directed to some other morally worthwhile good, but so that others may profit and sometimes profit generously. Matthew Wynia et al. found that a number of physicians felt that they would be more comfortable rationing if they could be assured that the money saved on the care of one patient would go back into patient care.[30] Although the distinction between an open and closed system is morally significant, there are moral problems even given a closed system. For example, the question about whether adequate resources are made available for health care in the first place can be framed in moral terms. But private, for-profit insurance also seems incompatible with the moral demands of insurance that aims at equality. As Thomas Bodenheimer underscores, for-profit, private insurance is based on dividing the population into higher- and lower-risk pots and requires the higher risk (sicker and older) to pay more for their care.[31] For some people, this will result in either no insurance or inadequate insurance.

Although a full analysis of this question is not within the scope of this book, we need to be mindful of the possibility that for-profit medical insurance is at odds with social capital, especially in the context of scarce medical resources, whether scarce by choice or because of the nature of the good. When profit is combined with the denial of beneficial care, people may experience it very differently than when profit is simply the silver lining of delivering care, as it may have been in some fee-for-service plans. Of course, the more frivolous the object on which the 'savings' are spent, the more likely it will seem that the patient is not receiving care because he is uncared for. This, in turn, challenges our reservoirs of trust and social capital. For now, we shall have to remain content with band-aid measures of the sort I mention. Although such measures may contribute to the conservation of social capital, they will not maximize it.

Notes

1 K. Levit et al. Health Spending Rebound Continues in 2002. *Health Affairs,* 2004; 23: 148.
2 C. DeNavas-Walt et al. Income, Poverty, and Health Insurance Coverage in the United States: 2003. *Current Population Reports of U.S. Census Bureau,* Department of Commerce Economics, and Statistics Administration, August 2004, pp. 60–226.
3 J.R. Gabel et al. Job-based health insurance in 2000: Premiums rise sharply while coverage grows. *Health Affairs* 2000; 19: 243–51.
4 The White House. *Fact Sheet: Guidance Released on Health Savings Accounts (HSAs),* Office of the Press Secretary, 22 December 2003, online, available at: <www.whitehouse.gov/news> (Accessed 15 September 2004).
5 *Kentucky Association of Health Plans v. Miller,* 123 S. Ct. 1471, 2003.
6 *Aetna Health, Inc. v. Davila,* 124 S. Ct. 2488, 2004.
7 I. Kawachi. Social Cohesion and Health. In *The Society and Population Health Reader: A State and Community Perspective,* Vol. 2, ed. A.R. Tarlov and R.F. St Peter. New York: The Free Press, 2000, p. 57; L.F. Berkman. Social Networks and Health: The Bonds that Heal, ibid., pp. 259–77.
8 H. Green. Health Insurers Face the Heat. *Best's Review,* March 2003, p. 12.
9 M. Ahern and M. Hendryx. Social Capital and Trust in Providers. *Social Science and Medicine,* 2003; 57: 1195–203.
10 M.A. Hall et al. Trust in Physicians and Medical Institutions: What is it, Can it be Measured, and Does it Matter? *Milbank Quarterly,* 2001; 79: 613–39.
11 See Community Policing Consortium. Online, available at: <http://www.communitypolicing.org>.
12 D.W. Brock. Broadening the Bioethics Agenda. *Kennedy Institute of Ethics Journal,* 2002; 10: 21–38; D. Callahan. Ends and Means: The Goods of Health Care. In *Ethical Dimensions of Health Policy,* ed. M. Davis et al. New York: Oxford University Press, 2002, pp. 3–18.
13 D. Mechanic. Models of Rationing: Professional Judgment and the Rationing of Medical Care, 140 *University of Pennsylvania Law Review* 1713, May 1992.

14 Institute of Medicine. *To Err is Human: Building a Safer Health System*, ed. L. Kohn et al., eds. Washington, DC: National Academy Press, 1999.

15 A. Whitman et al. How do Patients Want Physicians to Handle Medical Mistakes? A Survey of Internal Medicine Patients in an Academic Setting. *Archives of Internal Medicine*, 1996; 156: 2565–9; L. Leape. Error in Medicine. *Journal of the American Medical Association*, 1994; 272: 1851–7.

16 J.S. Mill. *On Liberty*. Cambridge, UK: Hackett Publishing Company, 1978.

17 J.A. Strausbaugh. It's Enough to Make You Sick: The Issue of Runaway Health Insurance has Made Lancaster Employers Feverish for Solutions. *Sunday News Lancaster*, PA, 21 April 2002, D-1.

18 DeNavas-Walt et al., op. cit., p. 14.

19 M.L. Lassey et al. *Health Care Systems Around the World*. Upper Saddle River, NJ: Prentice Hall Press, 1997, p. 220.

20 R.J. Blendon et al. Inequities in Health Care: A Five-Country Survey. *Health Affairs*, 2002; 21: 185.

21 Ibid., p. 188.

22 C. Krauss. Canada Looks for Ways to Fix Its Health Care System. *New York Times*, 12 September 2004, Section: International.

23 M. Kirby. Some Points that Hold Promise for a Deal. *Globe and Mail*, 14 September 2004, p. A5.

24 B. Laghi et al. PM Pulls Out a Deal. *Globe and Mail*, 16 September 2004, p. A1.

25 S. Stevens. Reform Strategies For The English NHS. *Health Affairs*, 2004; 23: 38.

26 Ibid.

27 Stevens, op. cit., p. 39.

28 Stevens, op. cit., p. 40.

29 L. Fleck and H. Squier. Facing the Ethical Challenges of Managed Care. *Family Practice Management*, 1995; October: 49–55; N. Daniels. Why Saying 'No' to Patients in the U.S. is So Hard: cost containment, Justice and Provider Autonomy. *The New England Journal of Medicine*, 1986; 314: 1381–3.

30 M. Wynia, e-mail correspondence, 28 December 2002.

31 T. Bodenheimer. The Movement for Universal Health Insurance: Finding Common Ground. *American Journal of Public Health*, 2003; 93: 112–15.

Bibliography

Ahern, M. and M. Hendryx. Social Capital and Trust in Providers. *Social Science and Medicine*, 2003; 57: 1195–203.

Altman, D. and L. Levitt. The Sad History of Health Care Cost Containment as Told in One Chart. *Health Affairs*, 23 January 2002, web exclusive W83. Online, available at: <http://www.healthaffairs.org>.

American Medical Association. *Managing Managed Care in the Medical Practice*. Norcross, GA: Coker Publishing, 1996.

American Medical Association Council on Ethical and Judicial Affairs. *Code of Medical Ethics Current Opinions and Annotations 8.13 (2)(b)*. Chicago: AMA, 2002–2003.

American Medical Association Council on Ethical and Judicial Affairs. *Code of Medical Ethics Current Opinions and Annotations 10.02*. Chicago: AMA Press, 2002.

American Nursing Association. Nursing's Social Policy Statement. Washington, DC: American Nurses Publishing, 1995. In J. Reitter-Teital. The Impact of Restructuring Professional Nursing Administration. *Journal of Nursing Administration*, 2002; 32, No. 1: 31–41.

Anderson, G.F. et al. It's the Prices, Stupid: Why the United States is So Different From Other Countries. *Health Affairs*, 2003; 22, No. 3: 103.

Angell, M. Medicine: The Endangered Patient-Centered Ethic. *Hastings Center Report*, February 1987.

Angell, M. and J.P. Kassirer. Quality and the Medical Marketplace—Following Elephants. *New England Journal of Medicine*, 1996; 335, No. 12: 883–5.

Applbaum, A.I. *Ethics for Adversaries*. Princeton: Princeton University Press, 1999.

Arrow, K. Uncertainty and the Welfare Economics of Medical Care. *American Economic Review*, 1963; LIII, No. 5: 851–83.

Backlund, E. et al. The Shape of the Relationship Between Income and Mortality in the United States: Evidence from the National Longitudinal Mortality Study. *Annals of Epidemiology*, 1996; 6: 12–20.

Baker, D.W. et al. Lack of Health Insurance and Decline in Overall Health in Late Middle Age. *New England Journal of Medicine*, 2001; 345, No. 15: 1106–12.

Barber, B. *The Logic and Limits of Trust*. New Brunswick, NJ: Rutgers University Press, 1983.

Beauchamp, T.L. Manipulative Advertising. In *Ethical Theory and Business*, 5th edn, ed. T.L. Beauchamp and N.E. Bowie. Upper Saddle River, NJ: Simon & Schuster, 1997, 472–80.

Belluck, P. Doctors' New Practices Offer Deluxe Service for Deluxe Fee. *New York Times*, 15 January 2002, Sec. A1.

Benjamin, M. Lay Obligations in Professional Relations. *Journal of Medicine and Philosophy*, 1985; 10, No. 1: 85–103.

Bergman, R. Study: Employers Consider Cost Over Quality in Health Purchases. *Hospitals and Health Networks*, 1994; 68, No. 5: 54.

Berk, M.L. and A.C. Monheit. The Concentration of Health Care Expenditures, Revisited. *Health Affairs*, 2001; 20, No. 2: 9–18.

Berkman, L.F. The Changing and Heterogeneous Nature of Aging and Longevity. *Annual Review of Gerontology and Geriatrics*, 1988; 8: 37–68.

Berkman, L.F. The Role of Social Relations in Health Promotion. In *The Society and Population Health Reader: Income Inequality and Health*, Vol. 1, ed. I. Kawachi et al. New York: New Press, 1999, 171–83.

Berkman, L.F. Social Networks and Health: The Bonds that Heal. In *The Society and Population Health Reader: A State and Community Perspective*, Vol. 2. ed. A.R. Tarlov and R.F. St Peter. New York: The Free Press, 2000.

Berkman, L.F. and S.L. Syme. Social Networks, Host Resistance and Mortality: a Nine Year Follow-up Study of Alameda County Residents. *American Journal of Epidemiology*, 1979; 109: 186–204.

Berlin, I. Two Concepts of Liberty. In *Liberalism and its Critics*, ed. M. Sandel. New York: University Press, 1984.

Black's Law Dictionary. 6th edition. St Paul: West Publishing Co., 1990.

Blazer, D.G. Social Support and Mortality in an Elderly Community Population. *American Journal of Epidemiology*, 1982; 115, No. 5: 684–94.

Blendon, R.J. and J.M. Benson. Americans' Views on Health Policy: A Fifty-Year Historical Perspective. *Health Affairs* 20, 2001; No. 2: 40.

Blendon, R.J. et al. Understanding the Managed Care Backlash. *Health Affairs*, 1998: 17, No. 4: 80–110.

Blendon, R.J. et al. Inequities in Health Care: A Five-Country Survey. *Health Affairs*, 2002; 21: 182–91.

Bloche, M.G. Fidelity and Deceit at the Bedside. *Journal of the American Medical Association*, 2000; 283, No. 14: 1881–3.

Bloche, M.G. Look Out! That's the Wrong Way to Patients' Rights. *Washington Post*, 22 July 2001, Sec. B02.

Bloche, M.G. and P.D. Jacobsen. The Supreme Court and Bedside Rationing. *Journal of the American Medical Association*, 2000; 284, No. 21: 2776–9.

Bodenheimer, T. The HMO Backlash—Righteous or Reactionary? *New England Journal of Medicine*, 1996; 335, No. 21: 1601–4.

Bodenheimer, T. The American Healthcare System—The Movement for Improved Quality in Health Care. *New England Journal of Medicine*, 1999; 340: 488–92.

Bodenheimer, T. The Movement for Universal Health Insurance: Finding Common Ground. *American Journal of Public Health*, 2003; 93, No. 1: 112–15.

Bodenheimer, T. and K. Sullivan. How Large Employers are Shaping the Health Care Marketplace. *New England Journal of Medicine*, 1998; 338, No. 14: 1003–8.

Bok, S. *Lying*. London: Quartet Books Limited, 1978.

Branch, W.T. Is the Therapeutic Nature of the Patient–Physician Relationship Being Undermined? A Primary Care Physician's Perspective. *Archives of Internal Medicine*, 2000; 160, No. 15: 2257–60.

Brenkert, G. Marketing Trust: Barriers and Bridges. *Business and Professional Ethics Journal*, 1997; 16, No. 1–3: 77–98.

Brenkert, G. Trust, Morality, and International Business. *Business Ethics Quarterly*, 1998; 8, No. 2: 293–317.

Brennan, T.A. An Ethical Perspective on Health Care Insurance Reform. *American Journal of Law and Medicine*, 1993; 19, No. 1 & 2: 37–74.

Brennan, T.A. Luxury Primary Care—Market Innovation or Threat to Access? *New England Journal of Medicine*, 2002; 346, No. 15: 1165–8.

Brett, A.S. The Case Against Persuasive Advertising by Health Maintenance Organizations. *New England Journal of Medicine*, 1992; 326, No. 20: 1353–6.

Brock, D.W. Broadening the Bioethics Agenda. *Kennedy Institute of Ethics Journal*, 2000; 10, No. 1: 21–38.

Bruhn, J. and S. Wolfe. *The Roseto Story: An Anatomy of Health*. Norman, OK: Oklahoma University Press, 1979.

Buchanan, A. Trust in Managed Care Organizations. *Kennedy Institute of Ethics Journal*, 2000; 10, No. 3: 189–212.

Bureau of Labor Statistics. Union Members Summary. United States Department of Labor, Washington, DC, 25 February 2003. Online, available at: <http://www.bls.gov/news.release/union2.nr0.htm.>

Bursztajn, H.J. More Law and Less Protection: 'Critogenesis,' 'Legal Iatrogenesis' and Medical Decision Making, *Journal of Geriatric Psychiatry*, 1985; 18, No. 2: 143–53.

Callahan, D. Ends and Means: The Goods of Health Care. In *Ethical Dimensions of Health Policy*, ed. M. Davis et al. Churchill, New York: Oxford University Press, 2002, 3–18.

Carr, A.Z. Is Business Bluffing Ethical? In *Ethical Theory and Business*, 5th edn, ed. T.L. Beauchamp and N.E. Bowie. New Jersey: Prentice Hall, 1997, 451–6.

Carson, T. Second Thoughts About Bluffing. In *Ethical Theory and Business*, 5th edn, ed. T.L. Beauchamp and N.E. Bowie. New Jersey: Prentice Hall, 1997, 456–462.

Case, R.B. et al. Living Alone After Myocardial Infarction. *Journal of the American Medical Association*, 1992; 267: 515.

Chernew, M. et al. Managed Care and Medical Technology: Implications for Cost Growth. *Health Affairs*, 1997; 16, No. 2: 202–3.

Chernew, M. et al. Managed Care, Medical Technology, and Health Care Cost Growth: A Review of the Evidence. *Medical Care, Research and Review*, 1998; 55, no. 3: 259–97.

Chervenak, F. et al. Responding to the Ethical Challenges Posed by the Business Tools of Managed Care in the Practice of Obstetrics and Gynecology. *American Journal of Obstetrics and Gynecology*, 1996; 175, No. 3: 523–7.

Chinba-Martine, M.A. and T.A. Brennan. The Critical Role of ERISA in State Health Reform. *Health Affairs*, 1994; 13, No. 2: 146.

Christensan, K.T. Ethically Important Restrictions Among Managed Care Organizations. *Journal of Law, Medicine and Ethics*, 1996; 23: 223–9.

Christianson, J.B. The Role of Employers In Community Healthcare Systems. *Health Affairs*, 1998: 7, No. 4: 163.

Clancy, C.M. and H. Brody. Managed Care: Jekyll or Hyde? *Journal of the American Medical Association*, 1995; 273, No. 4: 338–9.

Clark, R.C. Agency Costs Versus Fiduciary Duties. In *Principles and Agents: The Structure of Business*, ed. W. Pratt and R.J. Zeckhauser. Boston: Harvard Business School Press, 1985.

CNN.com. G.E. Workers Strike Over Health Care Costs. 14 January 2003. Online, available at: <http://www.cnn.com> (accessed 2003).

Coleman, J.S. Social Capital in the Creation of Human Capital. *American Journal of Sociology*, 1988; 94 (Suppl.): S95–S120.

Cooper, P.F. and B.S. Schone. More Offers, Fewer Takers for Employment Based Health Insurance 1987–1997. *Health Affairs*, 16, No. 6: 144.

Corbin, A.L. *Corbin on Contracts*. St. Paul: West Publishing Company: 1952.

Cropper, C.M. The Take-Charge Patient: Now You and Your Physician Can Be Partners. That's Healthier for Everyone. *Businessweek*, 26 August 2002, Issue #3796, 154.

Cunningham, P.J. et al. Do Consumers Know How Their Health Plan Works. *Health Affairs*, 2001; 20, No. 2: 159–66.

Daniels, N. Why Saying 'No' to Patients in the U.S. is So Hard: Cost Containment, Justice and Provider Autonomy. *New England Journal of Medicine*, 1986; 314: 1381–3.

Daniels, N. et al. Justice, Health and Health Policy. In *Ethical Dimensions of Health Policy*, ed. M. Davis et al. New York: Oxford University Press, 2002, 19–47.

Davies, H. et al. Public Disclosure of Performance Data: Does the Public Get What the Public Wants? *The Lancet*, 1999; 353, No. 9165: 1639–40.

Davis, K. et al. Choice Matters: Enrollees' Views of Their Health Plans. *Health Affairs*, 1995; 14, No. 2: 99–112.

Daynard, R. Regulating Tobacco: The Need for a Public Health Judicial Decision-Making Canon, *The Journal of Law, Medicine and Ethics*, 2002; 30: 281–9.

Declaration of Alma Atta. International Conference on Primary Health Care, Alma-Ata, U.S.S.R., 6–12 September 1978.

DeNavas-Walt, C. et al. Income, Poverty, and Health Insurance Coverage in the United States: 2003, Current Population Reports of U.S. Census Bureau Department of Commerce Economics, and Statistics Administration, August 2004.

Diderichsen, F. et al. The Social Basis of Disparities in Health. In *Social Epidemiology*, ed. I. Kawachi and L. Berkman. New York: Oxford University Press, 2000, 13–23.

Doescher, M.P. et al. Racial and Ethnic Disparities in Perceptions of Physician Style and Trust. *Archives of Family Medicine*, 2000; 9, No. 10: 1156–63.

Donelan, K. et al. The Cost of Health System Change: Public Discontent in Five Nations. *Health Affairs*, 1999; 18, No. 3: 206–16.

Dudley, R.A. et al. The Impact of Financial Incentives on Quality of Health Care. *Milbank Quarterly*, 1998; 76, No. 4: 649–86.

Duggan, D. Let's Keep Sex Behind Closed Doors. *Newsday*, 15 November 1998, Queens Edition.

Durkheim, E. *Suicide: A Study in Sociology*, ed. G. Simpson, trans. J.A. Spaulding and G. Simpson. New York: Free Press, 1951. As quoted in I. Kawachi and L. Berkman. Social Cohesion, Social Capital, and Health. In *Social Epidemiology*, ed. I. Kawachi and L. Berkman. New York: Oxford University Press, 2000.

Dworkin, R. The Model of Rules, In *Taking Rights Seriously*. Cambridge, MA: Harvard University Press, 1978.

EBRI Issue Brief # 193. Implications of ERISA for Health Benefits and the Number of Self-Funded ERISA Plans, January 1998. Online, available at: <http://www.ebri.com>.

EBRI Issue Brief # 253. Small Employers and Health Benefits: Findings from the 2002 Small Employer Health Benefits Survey, January 2003. Online, available at <www.ebri.com>.

Eddy, D.M. Benefit Language. *Journal of the American Medical Association*, 1996; 275, No. 8: 650–7.

Ekman, P. *Telling Lies*. New York: W.W. Norton and Co. Inc., 1992.

Ellis, S.J. Rationing: Fidelity and Stewardship are Incompatible When Attempted by Same Individual. *British Medical Journal*, 1999; 318, No. 7188: 941.

Emanuel, E.J. and N.N. Dubler. Preserving the Physician–Patient Relationship in the Era of Managed Care. *Journal of the American Medical Association*, 1995; 273, No. 4: 323–9.

Emanuel, E.J. and N.N. Dubler. Preserving the Physician–Patient Relationship in the Era of Managed Care. In *Contemporary Issues in Bioethics,* 5th edn. ed. T.L. Beauchamp and L. Walters. Belmont, CA: Wadsworth Publishing Company, 1999, 389–99.

Employers' Premium Costs to Rise 15 percent. *Managed Care Week*, 2003; 13, No. 1.

Enthoven, A.C. and S. Singer. The Managed Care Backlash and the Task Force in California. *Health Affairs*, 1998; 17, No. 4: 95–110.

Enthoven, A.C. et al. Consumer Choice and The Managed Care Backlash. *American Journal of Law and Medicine*, 2001; 27, No. 1: 1–15.

Ewen, S. *PR! A Social History of Spin*. New York: Basic Books, 1996.

Feldman, R.S. et al. Self-presentation and Verbal Deception: Do Self-Presenters Lie More? *Journal of Basic and Applied Social Psychology*, 2002; 24, No. 2: 163–70.

Fiscella, K. et al. Inequality in Quality: Addressing Socioeconomic, Racial, and Ethnic Disparities in Health Care. *Journal of the American Medical Association*, 2000; 283, No. 19: 2579–84.

Fleck, L. and H. Squier. Facing the Ethical Challenges of Managed Care. *Family Practice Management*, 1995; October: 49–55.

Fox, D.M. The Politics of Trust in American Health Care. In *Ethics, Trust, and the Professions*, ed. E. Pellegrino et al. Washington, DC: Georgetown University Press: 1991, 3–22.

Frankena, W. *Ethics,* 2nd edn. Englewood Cliffs, NJ: Prentice Hall, 1973.

Freeman, V.G. et al. Lying for Patients: Physician Deception of Third Party Payers. *Archives of Internal Medicine*, 1999; 159, No. 19: 2263–70.

Freudenheim, M. HMOs Cope with a Backlash on Cost Cutting. *New York Times*, 19 May 1996, Sec. 1.

Friedman, E. Money Isn't Everything: Nonfinancial Barriers to Access. *Journal of the American Medical Association*, 1994; 271, No. 19: 1535–38.

Fronstin, P. Employment-Based Health Benefits: Trends and Outlook. *EBRI Issues Brief #233*, 2001. Online, available at: <http://www.ebri.com>.

Fronstin, P. Sources of Health Insurance. *EBRI Issues Brief # 252* (2002). Online, available at <http://www.ebri.com>.

Fukuyama, F. *Trust: The Social Virtues and the Creation of Prosperity*. New York: The Free Press, 1995.

Furrow, B.R. The Problem of Medical Misadventures: A Review of E. H. Morreim's Holding Health Care Accountable. *Journal of Law, Medicine, and Ethics*, 2001; 29, No. 3–4: 381–95.

Furrow, B.R. et al. *Health Law: Cases Materials and Problems*. St Paul: West Publishing Co., 1997.

Gabel, J.R. et al. Job-Based Health Insurance in 2000: Premiums Rise Sharply While Coverage Grows. *Health Affairs*, 2000; 19, No. 5: 144–51.

Gabel, J.R. et al. Trends in Out-of-Pocket Spending by Insured American Workers 1990–1997. *Health Affairs*, 2001; 20, No. 2: 47–56.

Gabel, J.R. et al. Job-Based Health Insurance in 2001: Inflation Hits Double Digits, Managed Care Retreats. *Health Affairs*, 2001; 20, No. 5: 180–6.

Gabel, J.R. et al. Job-based Benefits in 2002: Some Important Trends. *Health Affairs*, 2002; 21, no. 5: 143–51.

Gabel, J.R. et al. Health Benefits in 2004: Four Years of Double-Digit Premium Increases Take Their Toll On Coverage. *Health Affairs*, 2004; 23, No. 5: 200–9.

Gallagher, T.H. et al. Patients' Attitudes Toward Cost Control Bonuses for Managed Care Physicians. *Health Affairs*, 2001; 20, No. 2: 186–92.

Gawande, A.A. et al. Does Dissatisfaction with Health Plans Stem From Having No Choices? *Health Affairs*, 1998; 17, No. 5: 184–94.

G.E. Workers Strike Over Health Care Costs. Online available at <http://www.cnn.com>, 14 January 2003.

Gediman, H.K. and J.S. Lieberman. *The Many Faces of Deceit*. New Jersey: Jason Aronson Inc., 1996.

Gilson, L. Trust and the Development of Health Care as a Social Institution. *Social Science and Medicine*, 2003; 56, No. 7: 1453–68.

Goold, S. Dorr. Money and Trust: Relationships between Patients, Physicians, and Health Plans. *Journal of Health Politics, Policy and Law*, 1998; 23, No. 4: 687–95.

Gostin, L.O. *Public Health Law*. Berkeley, CA and New York: University of California Press and Milbank Fund, 2000.

Gray, B.H. Trust and Trustworthy Care in the Managed Care Era. *Health Affairs*, 1997; 16, No. 1: 34–49.

Green, M. Managed Choice. *Best's Review*, March 2003; 71–6.

Greenfield, S. et al. Expanding Patient Involvement in Care: Effects on Patient Outcomes. *Annals of Internal Medicine*, 1985; 102: 520–8.

Greenfield, S. et al. Patients' Participation in Medical Care: Effects on Blood Sugar Control and Quality of Life in Diabetes. *Journal of General Internal Medicine*, 1988; 3: 448–57.

Grumbach, K. et al. Resolving the Gatekeeper Conundrum: What Patients Value in Primary Care and Referrals to Specialists. *Journal of the American Medical Association*, 1999; 282, No. 3: 261–6.

Guy, M. Policy Watch: Physicians and Patients Versus HMOs. *American Journal of Medicine*, 1996; 101, No. 5: 1.

Haggling with Health Care Providers about their Prices likely to Increase Sharply as Out-of-Pocket Costs Rise. H. Taylor and R. Leitman, eds., *Harris Interactive Healthcare News*, 2002; 2(5). Online available at: <http://www.harrisinteractive.com/news/newsletters_healthcare.asp>.

Hall, M.A. Healthcare Cost Containment and the Stratification of Malpractice Law. *Jurimetrics*, 1990; 30, No. 4: 501–9.

Hall, M.A. Informed Consent to Rationing Decisions. *The Milbank Quarterly*, 1993; 71, No. 4: 645–67.

Hall, M.A. Trust, Law and Medicine. *Stanford Law Review*, 2002; 55: 463–527.

Hall, M.A. et al. Trust in Physicians and Medical Institutions: What Is It, Can It be Measured, and Does It Matter? *Milbank Quarterly*, 2001; 79, No. 4: 613–39.

Hall, M.A. et al. How Disclosing HMO Physician Incentives Affects Trust. *Health Affairs*, 2002; 21, No. 2: 197–206.

Hampton, J.R. et al. Relative Contributions of History-Taking, Physical Examination, and Laboratory Investigation to Diagnosis and Management of Medical Outpatients. *British Medical Journal*, 1975; 2: 486–98.

Hardin, R. Street-Level Epistemology of Trust. *Politics and Society*, 1993; 21, No. 4: 506–8.

Hargraves, J. L. *Data Bulletin Number 17*. Washington, DC: Center for Studying Health System Change, 2000.

Harris Poll. 12–16 December 2003. In Many Happy with Health Insurance, Harris Poll Shows. *Heath Care Strategic Management*, 2003; 21, No. 3: 15.

Hart, J.T. Two Paths for Medical Practice. *The Lancet*, 1992; 340: 772–5.

Hart, J.T. and P. Dieppe. Caring Effects. *The Lancet*, 1996; 347: 1606–8.

Hasan, M. Let's End the Nonprofit Charade. *New England Journal of Medicine*, 1996; 334, No. 16: 1055–7.

Hause, J.S. et al. Social Relationships and Health. In *The Society and Population Health Reader: Income Inequality and Health*, Vol. 1, ed. I. Kawachi et al. New York: The New Press, 1999, 161–70.

Health of Nations: A Survey of Health-Care Finance. *The Economist*, 17 July 2004: 1–20.

Heffler et al. Health Spending Projections for 2002–2012. *Health Affairs*, Web Exclusive, 7 January 2003: W3 54–65.

Heffler et al. Health Spending Projections Through 2013. *Health Affairs*, Web Exclusive, 11 February 2004: W4 79–93.

Herbert, R. Torture by HMO. *New York Times*, 15 March 1996, Sec. A.

Hilfiken, D. Facing Our Mistakes. *New England Journal of Medicine*, 1984; 310: 118–22.

Hippocratic Corpus, The Physician, Decorum, XVI.

HMO Enrollment on the Decline; PPO's, POS Plans Gain in Membership and Satisfaction Ratings. *Employee Benefit Plan Review*, MA. 2001.

Hoffman, S. and M.C. Hatch. Stress, Social Support and Pregnancy Outcomes: A Reassessment Based on Recent Research. *Paediatric and Perinatal Epidemiology*, 1996; 10, No. 4: 380–405.

Holmes, O.W. *The Common Law*. Cambridge, Massachusetts: Belknap Press, 1967, at 1.

House, J.S. et al. Social Relationships and Health. In *The Society and Population Health Reader: Income Inequality and Health*, Vol. 1, ed. I. Kawachi et al. New York: New Press, 1999.

Iglehart, J.K. The American Health Care System-Expenditures. *New England Journal of Medicine*, 1999; 340, No. 1: 70–6.

Iglehart, J.K. Revisiting the Canadian Healthcare System. *New England Journal of Medicine*, 2000; 342, No. 26: 2007–12.

Iglehart, J.K. Changing Health Insurance Trends. *New England Journal of Medicine*, 2002; 347, No. 12: 956–62.

Illingworth, P. A Role for Stakeholder Ethics in Meeting the Ethical Challenges Posed by Managed Care Organizations. *HEC Forum*, 1999; 11, No. 4: 306–22.

Illingworth, P. Bluffing, Puffing, and Spinning in Managed-Care Organizations. *Journal of Medicine and Philosophy*, 2000; 25, No. 1: 62–76.

Institute of Medicine. *To Err is Human: Building a Safer Health System*, ed L. Kohn et al. Washington, DC: National Academy Press, 1999.

Institute of Medicine. President's Report to the Members. 16 October 2001, Annual Meeting. Online, available at: <http://www.iom.edu>.

Isaacs, S.L. Consumers' Information Needs: Results of a National Survey. *Health Affairs*, 1996; 15, No. 4: 31–41.

Jacobsen, P.D. *Strangers in the Night*. New York: Oxford University Press, 2002.

Jacobsen, P.D. and S. Pomfret. ERISA Litigation and Physician Autonomy. *Journal of the American Medical Association*, 283, 2000; No. 7: 921–6.

Jecker, N. Integrating Medical Ethics with Normative Theory: Patient Advocacy and Social Responsibility. *Theoretical Medicine*, 1990; 11: 125–39.

Jecker, N. Dividing Loyalties: Caring for Individuals and Populations. *Yale Journal of Health Policy, Law, and Ethics*, Spring 2001; 177.

Jenson, G.A. and M.A. Morrisey. Employer-Sponsored Health Insurance and Mandated Benefit Laws. *Milbank Quarterly* 1999; 77, No. 4: 425–59.

Jones, J. CMS Attacked over Delay in Reducing Secrecy. *British Medical Journal*, 2000; 321, No. 7254: 135.

Kahn, C. et al. Health Care for Black and Poor Hospitalized Medicare Patients. *Journal of the American Medical Association*, 1994: 271, No. 15: 1169–74.

Kaiser Family Foundation. National Survey of Consumer Experiences with Health Plans: Survey of Finding and Chartpack, June 2000.

Kaiser Family Foundation. *Kaiser Public Opinion Update*, August 2001.

Kaiser Family Foundation. Consumer Views of the Impact of Managed Care. In *Trends and Indicators in the Changing Medical Marketplace*, 2002.

Kaiser Family Foundation. *Chartbook: Trends and Indicators in the Changing Health Care Marketplace*, May 2002.

Kaiser Family Foundation. Kaiser Commission on Medicaid and the Uninsured Key Facts on Uninsured in America: Is Health Coverage Adequate? July 2002.

Kaiser Family Foundation. Kaiser Commission on Medicaid and the Uninsured Key Facts on The Uninsured and their Access to Health Care, January 2003.

Kaiser Family Foundation. *Chartbook: Trends and Indicators in the Changing Health Care Marketplace, 2004 Update*, April 2004.

Kaiser/Harvard PSRA Poll (22 August 1997). As described in R. Blendon et al. Understanding the Managed Care Backlash. *Health Affairs*, 17, No. 4: 80–110.

Kaiser Family Foundation/Harvard School of Public Health. National Survey of Consumer Experiences and Attitudes Toward Health Plans, August 2001.

Kaiser Family Foundation/Health Research and Educational Trust. *Employer Health Benefits 2004 Annual Survey*, September 2004.

Kao, A.C. et al. The Relationship Between Method of Physician Payment and Patient Trust. *Journal of the American Medical Association*, 1998; 280, No. 19: 1708–14.

Kao, A.C. et al. Patients' Trust in their Physicians: Effects of Choice, Continuity, and Payment Method. *Journal of General Internal Medicine*, 1998; 13: 681–6.

Kaplan, S.H. et al. Assessing the Effects of Physician–Patient Interaction on the Outcomes of Chronic Disease. *Medical Care*, 1989; 27: S5110–S5127.

Kassirer, J.P. The New Health Care Game. *New England Journal of Medicine*, 1996; 335, No. 6: 433.

Kassirer, J.P. Patients, Physicians, and the Internet. *Health Affairs*, 2000; 19, No. 6: 115–23.

Kaul, I. et al. (eds) *Global Public Goods*. New York: Oxford University Press. 1999.

Kawachi, I. Social Cohesion and Health. In *Society and Population Health Reader: A State and Community Perspective*, Vol. 2, ed A.R. Tarlov and R.F. St Peter. New York: The New Press, 2000, 57–74.

Kawachi, I. and L. Berkman. Social Cohesion, Social Capital, and Health. In *Social Epidemiology*, ed. L. Berkman and I. Kawachi. New York: Oxford University Press, 2000.

Kawachi, I., et al. Social Capital, Income Inequality and Mortality. In *The Society and Population Health Reader: Income Inequality and Health*, Vol. 1, ed. I. Kawachi et al. New York: New Press, 1999, 222–35.

Kawachi, I. et al. Introduction. In *The Society and Population Health Reader: Income Inequality and Health*, Vol. 1, ed. I. Kawachi et al. New York: The New Press, 1999, xi–xxxvi.

Kern, E.A., et al. The Influence of Gatekeeping and Utilization Review on Patient Satisfaction. *Journal of General Internal Medicine*, 1999; 14, No. 5: 287–96.

Kirby, M. Some Points that Hold Promise for a Deal. *Globe and Mail*, 14 September 2004, p. A5.

Knack, S. and P. Keefer. Does Social Capital Have an Economic Payoff? A Cross-Country Investigation. *Quarterly Journal of Economics*, 1997; 112 (4): 1252–5.

Krauss, C. Canada Looks for Ways to Fix Its Health Care System. *New York Times*, 12 September 2004, International Section.

Kronick, R. and T. Gilmer. Explaining the Decline in Health Insurance Coverage, 1979–1995. *Health Affairs*, 1999; 18, No. 2: 30–47.

Kumar, N. The Power of Trust in Manufacturer–Retailer Relationships. *Harvard Business Review* (November 1996): 92–106.

Kurlantzick, J. Liar, Liar. *Entrepreneur Magazine*, October 2003, pp. 68–71.

Kuttner, R. Must Good HMOs Go Bad? First of Two Parts: The Commercialization of Prepaid Group Health Care. *New England Journal of Medicine*, 1998; 338, No. 21: 1558–63.

Kuttner, R. The American Health Care System: Employer-Sponsored Health, Coverage. *New England Journal of Medicine*, 1999; 340, No. 3: 248–52.

La Porta, R. et al. Trust in Large Organizations. *AEA Papers and Proceedings*, 1997; 87, No. 2: 333–8.

Laghi, B. et al. PM Pulls Out a Deal. *Globe and Mail*, 16 September 2004, p. A1.

Landis, N.T. Internet Use Affects Health Care Decision-Making, Survey Confirms: Information Seekers Don't Divulge Personal Data. *American Journal of Health-System Pharmacy*, 2001; 58, No. 2: 103–8.

Lassey, M.L. et al. *Health Care Systems Around the World*. Upper Saddle River, NJ: Prentice Hall Press, 1997.

Leaffer, T. and B. Gonda. The Internet: An Underutilized Tool in Patient Education. *Computers in Nursing*, 2000 18, No. 1: 47–52.

Leape, L.L. Error in Medicine. *Journal of the American Medical Association*, 1994; 272, No. 23: 1851–7.

Levinsky, N.G. The Doctor's Master. *New England Journal of Medicine*, 1984; 311, No. 24: 1757.

Levinsky, N.G. Truth or Consequences. *New England Journal of Medicine*, 1998; 338, No. 13: 913–15.

Levit, K., et al. Inflation Spurs Health Spending in 2000. *Health Affairs*, 2002; 21, No. 1: 172–87.

Levit, K., et al. Trends In U.S. Health Care Spending, 2001. *Health Affairs*, 2003; 22, No. 1: 154–64.

Levit, K., et al. Health Spending Rebound Continues in 2002. *Health Affairs*, 2004; 23, No. 1: 147–59.

Lewis, S. A Guide to the Federal Patients' Bill of Rights Debate. Prepared for the Kaiser Family Foundation, August 2001.

Liar, Liar—the Pinocchio Dilemma. *Modern Physician*, August 1997, p. 6.

Love, M.M. et al. Continuity of Care and the Physician–Patient Relationship. *Journal of Family Practice*, 2000; 49, No. 11: 998–1004.

Lupton, D. et al. Caveat Emptor or Blissful Ignorance? Patients and the Consumerist Ethos. *Social Science and Medicine*, 1991; 33, No. 5: 559–68.

Macinko, J. and B. Starfield. The Utility of Social Capital in Research on Health Determinants. *Milbank Quarterly*, 2001; 79, No. 3: 387–427.

Maeder, T. Good Health is Just a Costly Way to Die. *Red Herring*, 1 September 2000, pp. 55–60.

Mariner, W.K. Problems with Employer-Provided Health Insurance—The Employee Retirement Income Security Act and Health Insurance and Health Care Reform. *New England Journal of Medicine*, 1992; 327, No. 23: 1683.

Mariner, W.K. Business v. Medical Ethics: Conflicting Standards for Managed Care. *Journal of Law, Medicine and Ethics*, 1995; 23: 236–46.

Mariner, W.K. Rationing Health Care and the Need for Credible Scarcity: Why Americans Can't Say No. *American Journal of Public Health*, 1995; 85, No. 10: 1439–45.

Marmot, M.G. et al. Contributions of Job Control and Other Social Variations in Coronary Heart Disease Incidence. *The Lancet*, 1997; 350, No. 9073: 235–9.

Martin, D.P. et al. Effect of a Gatekeeper Plan on Health Services Use and Changes: A Randomized Trial. *American Journal of Public Health*, 1989; 79: 1628–32.

Martin, J.A. and L.K. Bjerknes. The Legal and Ethical Implications of Gag Clauses in Physician Contracts. *American Journal of Law and Medicine*, 1996; 22, No. 4: 433–76.

Mashaw, J.L. and T.R. Marmor. Conceptualizing, Estimating and Reforming Fraud, Waste, and Abuse in Healthcare Spending. *Yale Journal on Regulation*, 1994; 11: 490.

Mays, G.P. et al. Managed Care Rebound? Recent Changes in Health Plans' Cost Containment Strategies. *Health Affairs*, Web Exclusive, 11 August 2004: W4 427–436.

McNamara, R. Capitation for Cardiologists: Accepting Risk for Coronary Artery Disease Under Managed Care. *American Journal of Cardiology*, 1998; 82, No. 10: 1178–82.

Mechanic, D. Models of Rationing: Professional Judgment and the Rationing of Medical Care. 140 *University of Pennsylvania Law Review*, May 1992, pp. 1713–54.

Mechanic, D. Dilemmas in Rationing Health Care Services: The Case for Implicit Rationing. *British Medical Journal*, 1995; 310, No. 6995: 1655–9.

Mechanic, D. Changing Medical Organization and the Erosion of Trust. *Milbank Quarterly*, 1996; 74, No. 2: 171–89.

Mechanic, D. The Functions and Limitations of Trust in the Provision of Medical Care. *Journal of Health Politics and Law*, 1998; 23, No. 4: 661–86.

Mechanic, D. Managed Care and the Imperative for a New Professional Ethic. *Health Affairs*, 2000; 19, No. 5: 100–12.

Mechanic, D. The Managed Care Backlash: Perceptions and Rhetoric in Health Care Policy and the Potential for Health Care Reform. *Milbank Quarterly*, 2001; 79, No. 1: 35–54.

Mechanic, D. and S. Meyer. Concepts of Trust Among Patients with Serious Illness. *Social Science and Medicine*, 2000; 51, No. 5: 657–68.

Mechanic, D. and M. Schlesinger. The Impact of Managed Care on Patients' Trust in Medical Care and Their Physicians. *Journal of the American Medical Association*, 1996; 275, No. 21: 1693–7.

Mechanic, D. and M. Schlesinger. Professionalism in Medicine: Can Patients Trust in Managed Care? *Journal of the American Medical Association*, 1996; 276, No. 12: 951.

Mill, J.S. *On Liberty*. Cambridge, UK: Hackett Publishing Company, 1978.

Mill, J.S. *Utilitarianism*, ed. O. Piest. Indiana: Bobbs-Merrill Educational Publishing, 1957.

Miller, R.H. and H.S. Luft. Does Managed Care Lead to Better or Worse Quality of Care? *Health Affairs*, 1997; 16, No. 5: 7–25.

Miller, R.H. and H.S. Luft. HMO Plan Performance Update: An Analysis of the Literature, 1997–2001. *Health Affairs*, 2002; 21, No. 4: 63.

Miller, T.E. and C.R. Horowitz. Disclosing Doctors' Incentives: Will Consumers Understand and Value the Information? *Health Affairs*, 2000; 19, No. 4: 149–55.

Miller T.E. and W.M. Sage. Disclosing Physician Financial Incentives. *Journal of the American Medical Association*, 1999; 281, No. 15: 1424–30.

Mills, R.J. Health Insurance Coverage: 2001. In *Current Population Reports*, U.S. Census Bureau, September 2002.

Milstead, J.A. Leapfrog Group: A Prince in Disguise or Just Another Frog? *Nursing Administration Quarterly*, 2002; 26: 16–25.

Mitchell, J.M., et al. Access to Bone Marrow Transplantation for Leukemia and Lymphoma: The Role of Sociodemographic Factors. *Journal of Clinical Oncology*, 1997; 15: 2644–51.

Montagne, C. Bargaining Health Benefits in the Workplace: An Inside View. *Milbank Quarterly*, 2002: 80, No. 3: 547–67.

Morreim, E.H. Redefining Quality by Reassigning Responsibility. *American Journal of Law and Medicine*, 1994; 20, No. 79: 79–104.

Morreim, E.H. *Balancing Act: The New Medical Ethics of Medicine's New Economics*. Washington, DC: Georgetown University Press, 1995.

Morreim, E.H. Moral Justice and Legal Justice in Managed Care: The Ascent of Contributive Justice. *Journal of Law, Medicine & Ethics*, 1995; 23: 247–65.

Morreim, E.H. Medicare Meets Resource Limits: Restructuring the Legal Standard of Care. 59 *University of Pittsburgh Law Review* 1, 1997, 28.

Morreim, E.H. *Holding Health Care Accountable*. New York: Oxford University Press, 2001.

Nelson, H. Non-Profit and For-Profit HMOs: Converging Practices but Different Goals? *Report of the Milbank Memorial Fund*, 1997, 18.

Newton, K. Social Capital and Democracy. *American Behavioral Scientist*, 1997; 40, No. 5: 575–86.

Novack D.H. et al. Physicians' Attitudes Toward Using Deception to Resolve Difficult Ethical Problems. *Journal of the American Medical Association*, 1998; 261, No. 20: 2980–5.

Nudelman, P.M. and L.M. Andrews. The 'Value-Added' of Not-For-Profit Health Plans [Sounding Board]. *New England Journal of Medicine*, 1996; 334, No. 16: 1057–9.

O'Brien, E. Employers' Benefits from Workers' Health Insurance. *Milbank Quarterly*, 2003; 81, No. 1: 5–43.

O'Brien, E. and J. Feder. Employment-Based Coverage and its Decline: The Growing Plight of Low-Wage Workers. Prepared for the Kaiser Commission on Medicaid and the Uninsured. Washington, DC: Henry J. Kaiser Foundation, May 1999.

OECD. OECD Health Data 2004—Frequently Requested Data. Online available at: <http://www.oecd.org>.

Ortho-Gomer, K. et al. Social Isolation and Mortality in Ischemic Heart Disease. *Acta Medical School*, 1988; 224: 205–15.

Parmet, W.E. Regulation and Federalism: Legal Impediments to State Health Care Reform. *American Journal of Law and Medicine*, 1993; XIX, Nos. 1 & 2: 132–6.

Parmet, W.E. After September 11: Rethinking Public Health Federalism. *Journal of Law, Medicine, and Ethics*, 2002; 30, No. 2: 201–12.

Pearson, S.D. and T. Hyams. Talking About Money: How Primary Care Physicians Respond to a Patient's Questions About Financial Incentives. *Journal of General Internal Medicine*, 2002; 17, No. 1: 75–8.

Peele, P.B. et al. Employer-Sponsored Health Insurance: Are Employers Good Agents for Their Employees? *Milbank Quarterly*, 2000; 78, No. 1: 5–21.

Pellegrino, E.D. Trust and Distrust in Professional Ethics. In *Ethics, Trust, and The Professions: Philosophical and Cultural Aspects*, ed. E.D. Pellegrino et al. Washington, DC: Georgetown University Press, 1991.

Peterson, E.D. et al. Racial Variation in the Use of Coronary Revascularization Procedures: Are the Differences Real? Do They Matter? *New England Journal of Medicine*, 1997; 336, No. 7: 480–6.

Pinker, S. Quebec Moves Toward Full Disclosure of Medical Errors. *CMAJ-JAMC*, 2002; 166, No. 6: 800.

Polzer, K. and P. Butler. Employee Health Plan Protections Under ERISA. *Health Affairs*, 1997; 16, No. 5: 93–102.

President's Commission for the Study of Ethical Problems in Medicine and Biomedical and Behavioral Research. Securing Access to Health Care. From *Securing Access to Health Care*, Vol. 1. U.S. Government Printing Office, 1983. In *Contemporary Issues in Bioethics*, 5th edn, ed. T.L. Beauchamp and L. Walters. Belmont, CA: Wadsworth Publishing Company, 1999, 362–8.

Prosser, W. and W. Keeton. *Prosser and Keeton on the Law of Torts*, 5th edn. St Paul, Minn.: West Publishing Company, 1984.

Putnam, R. *Making Democracy Work: Civic Tradition in Modern Italy*. Princeton: Princeton University Press, 1993.

Putnam, R. Bowling Alone: America's Declining Social Capital. *Journal of Democracy*, 1995; 6, No. 1: 65–78.

Putnam, R. *Bowling Alone*. New York: Simon & Schuster, 2000.

Putnam, R. Bowling Together. *American Prospect*, 2002; 13, No. 3: 20–2.

Randal, L. et al. How Managed Care Can Be Ethical. *Health Affairs*, 2000; 20, No. 4: 43–56.

Rawls, J. Distributive Justice. In *J. Rawls Collected Papers*, ed. S. Freeman. Cambridge, MA: Harvard University Press, 1967.

Reuben, R.C. In Pursuit of Health. *ABA Journal*, 1996; 82: 55.

Rhodes, R. Trust and Transforming Medical Institutions. *Cambridge Quarterly of Healthcare Ethics*, 2000; 4, No. 2: 205.

Robinson, J.C. The Future of Managed Care Organization. *Health Affairs*, 1999; 18, No. 2: 10.

Robinson, J.C. The End of Managed Care. *Journal of the American Medical Association*, 2001; 285, No. 20: 2622–8.

Rodwin, M. *Medicine, Money & Morals: Physicians' Conflicts of Interest*. New York: Oxford University Press, 1993.

Rogers, G.B. Income and Inequality as Determinants of Mortality: An International Cross-Section Analysis. In *The Society and Population Health Reader: Income Inequality and Health*, Vol. 1, ed. I. Kawachi et al. New York: The New Press, 1999, 5–13.

Romano, M. Loophole Tied to Bizarre Case. *Modern Healthcare*, 19 August 2000, p. 10.

Romanow, R.J. A Message to Canadians. In *Building on Values: The Future of Health Care in Canada (Final Report of the Commission on the Future of Health Care in Canada)*, November 2002.

Rosenbaum, S. Managed Care and Patients' Rights (Editorial). *Journal of the American Medical Association*, 2003; 289, No. 7: 906–7.

Rosmer, F. et al. Disclosure and the Prevention of Medical Errors. *Archives of Internal Medicine*, 2000; 160, No. 14: 2089–92.

Rosner, D. and G. Markovitz. The Struggle over Employee Benefits: The Role of Labor in Influencing Modern Health Policy. *Milbank Quarterly*, 2003; 81, No. 1: 45–68.

Roter, D. and J. Hall. *Doctors Talking with Patients/Patients Talking with Doctors: Improving Communication in Medical Visits*. Westport, CT: Auburn House, 1992.

Ruberman, W. et al. Psychosocial Influences on Mortality After Myocardial Infarction. *New England Journal of Medicine*, 1984; 311: 552–9.

Sabin, J. The Second Phase of Priority Setting: Fairness as a Problem of Love and the Heart: A Clinician's Perspective on Priority Setting. *British Medical Journal*, 1998; 317, No. 7164: 1002–4.

Safran, D.G. and D.A. Taira. Linking Primary Care Performance to Outcomes of Care. *Journal of Family Practice*, 1998; 47: 213–20.

Saguaro Seminar: Civic Engagement in America. Social Capital Research: What is Social Capital? Online, available at: <http://www.ksg.harvard.edu/saguaro/primer.htm> (accessed 15 September 2004).

Samuel, T.W. et al. The next stage in the health care economy: aligning the interests of patients, providers, and third-party payers through consumer-driven health plans. *American Journal of Surgery*, 2003; 186: 117–24.

Sapolsky, H.M. Empire and the Business of Health Insurance. *Journal of Health Politics, Policy and Law*, 1991; 16, No. 4: 747–61.

Sapolsky, H.M. et al. Corporate Attitudes Toward Health Care Costs. *Milbank Memorial Fund Quarterly*, 1981; 59, No. 4: 570.

Schaeffer, L.D. and L.C. Volpe. Focusing on the Health Care Consumer. *Health Affairs*, 1999; 18, No. 2: 25–7.

Scott, R.A. and L. Aiken. Organizational Aspects of Caring. *Milbank Quarterly*, 1995; 73: 77–95.

Seeman, T.E. Social Ties and Health: The Benefits of Social Integration. *Annals of Epidemiology*, 1996; 6, No. 5: 442–51.

Shapiro, A.K. and E. Shapiro. Patient–Provider Relationships and the Placebo Effect. In *Behavioral Health*, ed. J.D. Matarazzo et al. New York: J. Wiley and Sons, 1984.

Sheldon, K.M. et al. What is Satisfying about Satisfying Events? Testing Ten Candidate Psychological Needs. *Journal of Personality and Social Psychology*, 2001; 80, No. 2: 325–39.

Shively, C.A. The Behavior and Physiology of Social Stress and Depression in Female Cynomolgus Monkeys. *Biological Psychiatry*, 1997; 41, No. 8: 871–82.

Short, R. Griffiths NHS Management Inquiry Report. Canadian House of Commons, Social Services Committee, 20 June 1984.

Shortell, S. et al. Physicians as Double Agents: Maintaining Trust in an Era of Multiple Accountabilities. *Journal of the American Medical Association*, 1998; 280, No. 12: 1102–8.

Silvers, A. Protecting the Innocents: People with Disabilities and Physician-Assisted Dying. *Western Journal of Medicine*, 1997; 166, No. 6: 407–9.

Simmons, M. For Newly Jobless, Insurance Options are Few. *New York Times Final Edition*, 18 December 2001, Sec. F01.

Simon, S.R. et al. Views of Managed Care—A Survey of Students, Residents, Faculty and Deans at Medical Schools in the United States. *New England Journal of Medicine*, 1999; 340, No. 12: 930.

Singer, P. *Writings on an Ethical Life*. New York: HarperCollins, 2000.

Slovich, P. Perceived Risk, Trust and Democracy. *Risk Analysis*, 1993; 13, No. 6: 675–82.

Smith, S. et al. The Next Ten Years of Health Spending: What Does the Future Hold? *Health Affairs*, 1998; 17, No. 5: 128–40.

Somerville, Margaret. *The Ethical Canary*. Toronto: Viking Press, 2000.

Sorbero, M.E. et al. The Effect of Capitation on Switching Primary Care Physicians. *HSR: Health Services Research*, 2003; 38, No. 1, Part 1.

Spencer, E. et al. (eds) *Organizational Ethics in Healthcare*. New York: Oxford University Press, 2000.

Spire, H. *The Power of Hope*. New Haven: Yale University Press, 1998.

Starr, P. *The Transformation of American Medicine*. New York: Basic Books, Inc., 1949.

Starr, P. *The Social Transformation of American Medicine*. New York: Basic Books Inc., 1982.

Stauffer, M. and D.R. Levy (eds) *State by State Guide to Managed Care Law*. New York: Aspen Publishers Inc., 2000.

Stephenson, J. Patient Pretenders Weave Tangled 'Web' of Deceit. *Journal of the American Medical Association*, 1998; 280, No. 15: 1297.

Stevens, S. Reform Strategies For The English NHS. *Health Affairs*, 2004; 23, No. 3: 37–44.

Stone, A.A. *Law, Psychiatry and Morality*. Washington, DC: APA Press, 1984.

Stone, A.A. Paradigms, Pre-emptions, and Stages: Understanding the Transformation of American Psychiatry by Managed Care. *International Journal of Law and Psychiatry*, 1995; 18, No. 4: 353–87.

Strausbaugh J.A. It's Enough to Make You Sick: The Issue of Runaway Health Insurance has Made Lancaster Employers Feverish for Solutions. *Sunday News Lancaster,* PA, 21 April 2002, Sec. D-1.

Studdert, D.M. and C.R. Gresenz. Enrollee Appeals of Preservice Coverage Denials at 2 Health Maintenance Organizations. *Journal of the American Medical Association,* 2003; 289, No. 7: 864–70.

Sulmasy, D.P. et al. Physicians' Ethical Beliefs About Cost-control Arrangements. *Archives of Internal Medicine,* 2000; 160, No. 5: 649–57.

Susznski, M. Brieflines, Health Insurers Feel the Heat. *Best's Review,* March 2003; 12.

Taylor, H. Harris Poll #38, 29 July 1998: Hostility to Managed Care Continues to Grow, But It Is Far From Overwhelming. Online, available at: <http://www.harrisinteractive.com/harris_poll/index.asp?PID=170>.

Taylor, H. and R. Leitman (eds) While Managed Care is Still Unpopular, Hostility Has Declined. *Health Care News,* 2002; 2, No. 20, 21 October.

Thom, D.H. Physician behaviors that predict patient trust. *Journal of Family Practice,* 2001; 50: 323–8.

Thom, D.H. and B. Campbell. Patient–Physician Trust: An Exploratory Study. *Journal of Family Practice,* 1997; 44, No. 2: 169–76.

Thorpe, K.E. et al. Why Are Workers Uninsured? Employer-Sponsored Health Insurance in 1997. *Health Affairs,* 1999; 18, No. 2: 213–18.

Treaster, J.B. Aetna Agreement With Doctors Envisions Altered Managed Care. *The New York Times,* 23 May 2000. Late Edition—Final, Section A, p. 1, Col. 1.

Turner, J. et al. The Importance of Placebo Effects in Pain Treatment and Research. *Journal of the American Medical Association,* 1994; 27, No. 20: 1609–14.

Tweed, V. Making HMOs Compete. *Business Health,* 1994; 12, No. 10: 27–38.

U.S.A. Today/CNN/Gallup Poll, 5–8 July 2002. As described in Jones, J.M. Poll Analyses: Americans Express Little Trust in CEOs of Large Corporations or Stockbrockers. *Gallup News Service,* 17 July 2002.

U.S. Census Bureau. *Current Population Survey.* Online, available at: <http://landview.census.gov/hhes/www/hlthin01.html> (30 May 2002).

U.S. Census Bureau. *Current Population Survey,* MA, 1999.

U.S. General Accounting Office. *Employment-Based Health Insurance: Costs Increase and Family Coverage Decreases* (GAO/ HEHS-97-35). Washington, DC: U.S. Government Printing Office, February 1997.

U.S. General Accounting Office. *Consumer Health Care Information: Many Quality Commission Recommendations Are Not Current Practice.* Washington, DC: General Accounting Office, 1998.

Useem, J. Should You Lie? *Fortune Small Business,* November 1999, 41.

Waldmann, R.J. Income Distribution and Infant Mortality. In *The Society and Population Health Reader: Income Inequality and Health,* Vol. 1, ed. I. Kawachi et al. New York: The New Press, 1999, 14–27.

Wallack, S.S. and C.P. Tompkins, Realigning Incentives in Fee-for-Service Medicare; a proposal to reform Medicare payment while retaining the fee-for service system, *Health Affairs,* 2003; 22: 59–70.

Weiss, L.J. and J. Blustein. Faithful Patients: The Effect of Long-Term Physician–Patient Relationships on the Costs and Use of Health Care by Older Americans. *American Journal of Public Health,* 1996; 86, No. 12: 1742–7.

Weiss, R. HMO Earnings Climb to $322 Million in First Quarter 2001. *Business Wire,* 26 November 2001.

Weston, B. and M. Lauria. Patient Advocacy in the 1990s. *New England Journal of Medicine*, 1996; 334, No. 8: 543–4.

White House, Fact Sheet: Guidance Released on Health Savings Accounts (HASs). Office of the Press Secretary, 22 December 2003. Online, available at: <www.whitehouse.gov/news> (accessed 15 September 2004).

Whitman, A. et al. How do Patients Want Physicians to Handle Medical Mistakes? A Survey of Internal Medicine Patients in an Academic Setting. *Archives of Internal Medicine*, 1996; 156, No. 22: 2565–9.

Wilkinson, R.G. Income Distribution and Life Expectancy. In *The Society and Population Health Reader: Income Inequality and Health*, Vol. 1, ed. I. Kawachi et al. New York: The New Press, 1999, 28–35.

Wilkinson, R.G. Social Relations, Hierarchy, and Health. In *The Society and Population Health Reader: Income Inequality and Health*. Vol. 1, ed. I. Kawachi et al. New York: The New Press, 1999, 211–35.

Williams, R.B. et al. Prognostic: Importance of Social and Economic Resources Among Medically Treated Patients with Angiographically Documented Coronary Heart Disease. *Journal of the American Medical Association*, 1992; 267: 520–4.

Wolfe, S. and J. Bruhn. *The Power of the Clan: A 25-year Prospective Study of Roseto, PA*. New Brunswick, NJ: Transaction Publishers, 1992.

Woolcock, M. Social Capital and Economic Development: Toward a Theoretical Synthesis and Policy Framework. *Theory and Society*, 1998; 27: 151–208.

Woolhandler, S. and D.U. Himmelstein. Extreme Risk—The New Corporate Proposition for Physicians. *New England Journal of Medicine*, 1995; 334, No. 16: 1706–9.

Wu, A.W. et al. How House Officers Cope with Their Mistakes. *Western Journal of Medicine*, 1993; 159: 5565–9.

Wu, A. et al. Quality of Care and Outcomes of Adults with Asthma Treated by Specialists and Generalists in Managed Care. *Archives of Internal Medicine*, 2001; 161, No. 21: 2554–60.

Wynia, M.K. et al. Physician Manipulation of Reimbursement Rules for Patients: Between a Rock and a Hard Place. *Journal of the American Medical Association*, 2000; 238, No. 14: 1858–65.

Young, D. Studies Show Drug Ads Influence Prescription Decisions, Drug Costs. *American Journal of Health-System Pharmacy*, 2002; 59, No. 1: 14, 16.

Zachry, W. et al. Relationship Between Direct-to-Consumer Advertising and Physician Diagnosing and Prescribing. *American Journal of Health-System Pharmacy*, 2002; 59, No. 1: 42–9.

Zaner, R.M. The Phenomenon of Trust and the Patient–Physician Relationship. In *Ethics, Trust, and the Professions: Philosophical and Cultural Aspects*, ed. E.D. Pellegrino et al. Washington, DC: Georgetown University Press, 1991.

Zheng, B. et al. Development of a Scale to Measure Patients' Trust in Health Insurers. *Health Services Research*, 2002; 37, No. 1: 187–202.

Legal Cases, Laws, and Statutes

Aetna Health, Inc. v. Davila, 124 S. Ct. 2488, 2004.

Backman v. Polaroid Corporation, 910 F. 2d 10 (1st Cir. 1990).

Bauman v. U.S. Healthcare, Inc. (In Re U.S. Healthcare) 193 F. 3d 151 (3d Cir. 1999).

Brief of Health Law, Policy and Ethics Scholars as Amici Curiae in Support of Respondents. *Pegram v. Herdrich*, 530 U.S. 211 (2000), (No. 98-1949).

Canterbury v. Spence, F.2d 772 (D.C. Cir. 1972).

Cicio v. Vytra Health Care, 321 F.3d 83 (2nd Cir. 2003).

Crum v. Health Alliance-Midwest Inc., 47 F. Supp. 2d 1013 (C.D. Ill. 1999).

Cruzan v. Director Missouri Department of Health, 497 U.S. 261 (1990).

Conn. Gen. Stat. 33-313(e) (West Supp. 1992).

Davis v. Virginia R.R. Co., 361 U.S. 354, 357 (1960).

Dodge v. Ford Motor Co., Supreme Court of Michigan, 204 Mich. 459, 170 N.W. 668 (1919).

Drolet v. Healthsource, 968 F. Supp., 757 (D.N.H. 1997).

Dukes v. U.S. Healthcare Inc. 57 F. 3d 350 (3d Cir. 1995).

Eddy v. Colonial Life Insurance Co. of AM., 919 F 2d 747, 750 (D. C. Cir. 1990).

The Employment Retirement Income Security Act of 1974, P.L. 93–406 88 Stat. 832, (1974) codified at 29 U.S.C. 1001 et seq. (2005).

Greenman v. Yuba, 59 Cal. 2d 57, 337 P. 2d 897, 27 Cal. Rptr. 697 (1962).

Guth v. Luft, 5A.2d 503, 510 (Del. Supr. 1939).

Herrera v. Lovelace Health Systems Inc., 35 F. Supp. 2d 1327 (D.M.N. 1999).

H.R. Rep. No. 533, 93d Cong., 1st Sess. 3 reprinted in 1974 U.S.C.C.A.N. 4639, 4642 (1973).

Kentucky Association of Health Plans v. Miller, 538 U.S. 329 (2003).

Lazorko v. Pennsylvania Hospital, 237 F. 3d 242 (3d Cir. 2000).

McClellan v. Health Maintenance Org. of Pennsylvania, 604 A. 2d 1053 (Pa. Supcr. Ct 1992).

McGann v. H & H Music Company, 742 F 392 (S.D. Tex. 1990) affirmed 946 F 2d 401 (5th Cir., 1991).

Moore v. The Regent of the University of California, 51 Cal. 3d 120 (1990).

Pegram v. Herdrich, 530 U.S. 211 (2000).

Preamble of Canada Health Act, R.S.C. 1985, c. C-6, Preamble.

Revised Model Business Code (4.01 9c).

Revised Model Business Code 858. 30 (a) (1992).

Rush Prudential HMO, Inc. v. Moran, 536 U.S. 355 (2002).

Shaw v. Delta Airlines Inc., 463 U.S. 815 (1983).

Shea v. Eisenstein 208 F. 3d 712 (8th Cir 2000).

Tarasoff v. Regents of the University of California, 131 Cal. Rptr. 14, 551 P. 2d 334 (Cal. 1976).

Texas Civ. Prac. & Rem. Code §88.002 (1999).

Tufino v. NY Hotel and Motel Trades Council, 646 NY S. 2d 799 (A.D. 1 Dept. 1996).

Varity Corp. v. Howe, 516 U.S. 489 (1996).

Ward v. Alternative Health Delivery System, 55 F. Supp. 2d 694, 699 (W.D. Ky. 2000).

Wickline v. State of California, 192 Cal. App 3d 1630 (1986).

Index